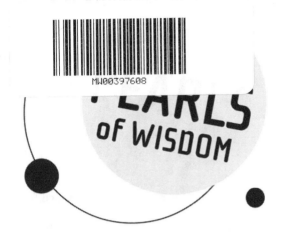

General Surgery
ABSITE AND BOARD REVIEW

Third Edition

Matthew J. Blecha, MD
Andrew Brown, MD

McGraw-Hill
Medical Publishing Division

New York Chicago San Francisco Lisbon London
Madrid Mexico City Milan New Delhi
San Juan Seoul Singapore
Sydney Toronto

The McGraw·Hill Companies

General Surgery ABSITE and Board Review, Third Edition

1 2 3 4 5 6 7 8 9 0   CUS/CUS   0 9 8 7 6 5

ISBN 0-07-146431-X

Notice

Medicine is an ever-changing science. As new research and clinical experience broaden our knowledge, changes in treatment and drug therapy are required. The authors and the publisher of this work have checked with sources believed to be reliable in their efforts to provide information that is complete and generally in accord with the standards accepted at the time of publication. However, in view of the possibility of human error or changes in medical sciences, neither the authors nor the publisher nor any other party who has been involved in the preparation or publication of this work warrants that the information contained herein is in every respect accurate or complete, and they disclaim all responsibility for any errors or omissions or for the results obtained from use of the information contained in this work. Readers are encouraged to confirm the information contained herein with other sources. For example and in particular, readers are advised to check the product information sheet included in the package of each drug they plan to administer to be certain that the information contained in this work is accurate and that changes have not been made in the recommended dose or in the contraindications for administration. This recommendation is of particular importance in connection with new or infrequently used drugs.

The editors were Catherine A. Johnson and Marsha Loeb.
The production supervisor was Phil Galea.
The cover designer was Handel Low.
Von Hoffmann Graphics was printer and binder.

This book is printed on acid-free paper.

Cataloging-in-Publication data for this title is on file at the Library of Congress.

EDITORS-IN-CHIEF:

Matthew J. Blecha, MD
Department of Surgery
St. Joseph Hospital
Chicago, IL

Andrew Brown, MD
Emergency Medicine Physician
St. Catherine's Hospital
East Chicago, IN

CONTRIBUTORS TO PREVIOUS EDITIONS:

"Pediatric Surgery"
William T. Adamson, MD
Pediatric Surgery Fellow
The Children's Hospital of Philadelphia
Philadelphia, PA

"Great Vessel Disease"
Beth A. Ballinger, MD
Assistant Professor of Vascular Surgery
The University of IA Hospitals & Clinics
Iowa City, IA

"Pharynx, Larynx, Mouth, Tongue, Jaw and Salivary Glands"
Dennis R. Banducci, MD
Associate Professor
Section of Plastic & Reconstructive Surgery
Hershey, PA

Gwenda Lyn Breckler, MD
Department of Surgery
Chicago Medical School
Mt. Sinai Hospital
Chicago, IL

"Great Vessel Disease"
"Venous and Lymphatic Disorders"
John D. Corson, MD, Ch.B, FRCS, FACS
Department of Surgery
The University of IA Hospitals & Clinics
Iowa City, IA

"Endocrine and Metabolic Response to Injury"
G. Paul Dabrowski, MD
Assistant Professor of Surgery
University of Pennsylvania
Philadelphia, PA

"ENT and Paranasal Sinus"
Dennis D. Diaz, MD
Assistant Professor of Surgery
Department of Otolaryngology-Head and Neck Surgery
Penn State/Geisinger Health Systems
Hershey, PA

"Thyroid and Parathyroid Glands"
Gerard M. Doherty, MD
Assistant Professor of surgery
Washington University
School of Medicine
St. Louis, MO

"Hemostasis, Bleeding Disorders, and Transfusions"
Ron M. Fairman, MD
Assistant Professor of Surgery
University of Pennsylvania
Philadelphia, PA

"Endocrine and Metabolic Response to Injury"
Seth Daniel Force, MD
Instructor in Surgery
University of Pennsylvania
Philadelphia, PA

"Mediastinum, Chest Wall, Lung, and Pleura"
Richard Freeman, MD
Section of General Thoracic Surgery
University of Washington
School of Medicine
Seattle, WA

"Neurosurgery"
Robert J. Gewirtz, MD
Assistant Professor of Neurosurgery
Department of Surgery
University of Kentucky
Chandler Medical Center
Lexington, KY

"Orthopedic Surgery"
John T. Gorczyca, MD
Assistant Professor
Division of Orthopedic Surgery
University of Kentucky
Chandler Medical Center
Lexington, KY

"Cutaneous Tissue"
Wesley Hall, MD
Division of Plastic & Reconstructive Surgery
Penn State/Geisinger Health System
Hershey, PA

"Cutaneous Tissue"
Randy M. Hauck, MD
Division of Plastic & Reconstructive Surgery
Penn State/Geisinger Health System
Hershey, PA

"Vascular Trauma"
"Diseases of the Peripheral Vessels"
Timothy C. Hodges, MD
Assistant Professor of Surgery
University of Missouri-Kansas City
School of Medicine
Kansas City, MO

"Liver Surgery"
Todd K. Howard, MD
Washington University
School of Medicine
St. Louis, MO

"Neurotology"
May Huang, MD
Assistant Professor
Neurotology & Otology
Penn State/Geisinger Health System
Hershey, PA

"Congenital Heart Disease"
Charles B. Huddleston, MD
Washington University
School of Medicine
St. Louis, MO

"Trauma"
Karen S. Hunter, MD
Assistant Professor
Division of Trauma/Critical Care
The University of Tennessee
Knoxville, TN

"Surgical Infections""Preoperative Preparation"
Kamal M.F. Itani, MD
Assistant Professor
Baylor College of Medicine
Associate Chief, Surgery
Chief, Ambulatory Surgery
Veterans Affairs Medical Center
Houston, TX

"Anesthesia"
Jeffrey S. Jacobs, MD
Assistant Professor of Anesthesiology
Miami VAMC/Jackson Memorial Hospital
University of Miami
Miami, FL

"Cardiac Surgery"
M. Salik A. Jahania, MD
Resident General Surgery
Post Doctoral Research Fellow
Department of Surgery
University of Kentucky
College of Medicine
Lexington, KY

"Pharynx, Larynx, Mouth, Tongue, Jaw and Salivary Glands"
Keith Jeffords, MD, D.D.S.
Resident
Section of Plastic & Reconstructive Surgery
Penn State/Geisinger Health Systems
Hershey, PA

"Appendix"
Walter Koltun, MD
Department of Surgery
Penn State/Geisinger Health Systems
Hershey, PA

"Head and Neck Surgery/Tumors"
Roger J. Levin, MD
Assistant Professor of Surgery
Section of Otolaryngology
Head and Neck Surgery
Penn State/Geisinger Health Systems
Penn State University
College of Medicine
Hershey, PA

"Intestinal Ischemia Disorders"
Walter Longo, MD
St. Louis University Medical Center
St. Louis, MO

"Neurosurgery Review"
Lloyd Maliner, MD
Section of Neurosurgery
Penn State/Geisinger Health Systems
Hershey, PA

"Gastrointestinal Surgery/Diseases"
"Fluid, Electrolyte and Nutritional Management"
Robert G. Martindale, MD, Ph.D.
Associate Professor of Surgery
Section of Gastrointestinal Surgery
Medical College of Georgia
Augusta, GA

Kimball I. Maull, MD
Director
The Trauma Center at Carraway
Carraway Methodist Medical Center
Birmingham, AL

"Congenital Heart Disease"
Eric N. Mendeloff, MD
Assistant Professor of Surgery
Washington University
School of Medicine
St. Louis, MO

"Esophageal Surgery"
Ravi Moonka, MD
Staff Surgeon
Puget Sound Veterans Affairs Medical Center
Department of Surgery
University of Washington Medical Center
Seattle, WA

"Pediatric Surgery"
Michael L. Nance, MD
Schnaufer Senior Surgical Fellow
The Children's Hospital of Philadelphia
Philadelphia, PA

"Abdominal Wall Hernias"
Prashant K. Narain, MD
Department of Surgery
Medical College of Virginia
Richmond, VA

"Venous and Lymphatic Disorders"
Munier Nazzal, MD, FRCS
Department of Surgery
The University of Iowa Hospitals & Clinics
Iowa City, IA

"Hemostasis, Bleeding Disorder, and
Transfusions"
David Neschis, MD
Department of Surgery
University of Pennsylvania
Philadelphia, PA

"Stomach"
"Eicosanoids in Surgery"
Juan B. Ochoa, MD
Assistant Professor
General Surgery
Section of Trauma & Critical Care
University of Kentucky
Lexington, KY

"Esophageal Surgery"
Carlos A. Pellegrini, MD
Professor and Chairman
Department of Surgery
University of Washington Medical Center
Seattle, WA

"Neurosurgery Review"
Stephen K. Powers, MD
Professor and Chief
Section of Neurosurgery
Penn State/Geisinger Health Systems
Hershey, PA

"Esophagus and Diaphragmatic Hernias"
Laurie Reeder, MD
Section of General Thoracic Surgery
School of Medicine
Seattle, WA

"Cardiac Surgery"
Juan A. Sanchez, MD
Assistant Professor
Department of Surgery
University of Kentucky
College of Medicine
Lexington, KY

"Abdominal Wall Hernias"
Jeannie F. Savas, MD
Department of Surgery
Medical College of Virginia
Richmond, VA

"Vascular Trauma"
"Diseases of the Peripheral Vessels"
William B. Schroder, MD
Chief, Section of Vascular Surgery
University of Missouri, Kansas City
Kansas City, MO

"Small Intestine"
Anthony J. Senagore, MD
Associate Professor of Surgery
Interim Program Director
General Surgery Residency
Butterworth Hospital
Michigan State University
Grand Rapids, MI

"Pediatric ENT"
Andrew Shapiro, MD
Department of Surgery
Penn State/Geisinger Health Systems
Hershey, PA

"Esophagus and Diaphragmatic Hernias"
"Mediastinum, Chest Wall, Lung and Pleura"
Eric Vallieres, MD
Section of General Thoracic Surgery
University of Washington
School of Medicine
Seattle, WA

"Stomach"
"Eicosanoids in Surgery
Boris Vinogradski, MD
Surgical Resident
Section of Trauma and Critical Care
University of Kentucky
Lexington, KY

"Esophagus and Diaphragmatic Hernias"
"Mediastinum, Chest Wall, Lund, and Pleura"
Douglas E. Wood, MD
Head, Section of General Thoracic Surgery
University of Washington
School of Medicine
Seattle, WA

"Thyroid and Parathyroid Glands"
John H. Yim, MD
Resident in General Surgery
Washington University
School of Medicine
St. Louis, MO

INTRODUCTION

Congratulations! *General Surgery ABSITE and Board Review: Pearls of Wisdom*, third edition, will help you improve your knowledge base in surgery. Originally designed as a study aid to improve performance on the Surgery Boards and ABSITE exams, this book is full of useful information. A few words are appropriate in discussing intent, format, limitations and use.

Since *General Surgery ABSITE and Board Review* is primarily intended as a study aid, the text is written in a rapid-fire question/answer format. This way, readers receive immediate gratification. Moreover, misleading or confusing "foils" are not provided. This eliminates the risk of erroneously assimilating an incorrect piece of information that makes a big impression. Questions themselves often contain a "pearl" intended to reinforce the answer. Additional "hooks" may be attached to the answer in various forms, including mnemonics, visual imagery, repetition, and humor. Additional information, not requested in the question, may be included in the answer. Emphasis has been placed on distilling trivia and key facts that are easily overlooked, quickly forgotten and that somehow seem to be needed on board examinations.

Many questions have answers without explanations. This enhances ease of reading and rate of learning. Explanations may often occur in a later question/answer. Upon reading an answer, the reader may think, "Hm, why is that?" or "Are you sure?" If this happens to you, go check! Truly assimilating these disparate facts into a framework of knowledge absolutely requires further reading of the surrounding concepts. Information learned in response to seeking an answer to a particular question is retained much better than information that is passively observed. Take advantage of this! Use this book with your preferred texts handy and open.

General Surgery ABSITE and Board Review risks accuracy by aggressively pruning complex concepts down to the simplest kernel—the dynamic knowledge base and clinical practice of medicine is not like that! Furthermore, new research and practice occasionally deviates from that which likely represents the right answer for test purposes. This text is designed to maximize your score on a test. Refer to your most current sources of information and mentors for direction for practice.

PLEASE NOTE:

> **The second and third editions of Pearls differs from the first in a few ways. Notably, facts most applicable to general surgeons have been highlighted. Excessive information pertaining to surgical subspecialties have been removed in attempt to highlight the features of those subspecialties most pertinent to ABSITE and board exams. Continuing in this light, questions which are felt to be especially high yield in studying for the general surgery in-service and board exams have had their question and answer italicized.**

This book is also designed to be re-used several times to allow memorization. A hollow bullet is provided for any scheme of keeping track of questions answered correctly or incorrectly.

We welcome your comments, suggestions and criticism. Great effort has been made to verify these questions and answers. Some answers may not be the answer you would prefer. Most often this is attributable to variance between original sources. Please make us aware of any errors you find. We hope to make continuous improvements and would greatly appreciate any input with regard to format, organization, content, presentation or about specific questions.

Study hard and good luck!

MJB & AB

TABLE OF CONTENTS

GENERAL PRINCIPLES PEARLS

The feasibility of an operation is not the best indication for its performance.
Henry, Lord of Cohen Birkenhead

○ **What is the most common site of infection in patients with diabetes mellitus (DM)?**

The urinary tract.

○ **What are the most common organisms isolated from diabetic foot ulcers?**

Gram positive cocci; however, infections are typically polymicrobial.

○ **What is the predictive value of a test?**

The percentage of positive results that are true positives.

○ **What are the manifestations of gastrointestinal autonomic neuropathy?**

Intractable diarrhea and steatorrhea.

○ **T/F: Hydralazine is a good choice for patients with neurogenic hypertension.**

False.

○ **How long do nonsteroidal anti-inflammatory drugs (NSAIDs) inhibit platelet function?**

Aspirin inhibits platelet function for the life of the platelet (7 days). Most other NSAIDs affect platelet function only while the drug has significant serum levels (i.e., 1 or 2 days).

○ **What is the diagnostic test of choice for detecting dysphagia in diabetic patients?**

Fiberoptic esophagoscopy with mucosal brushings and biopsy.

○ *Why are beta-blockers not used alone in the preoperative preparation of patients with a pheochromocytoma?*

Unopposed alpha stimulation may provoke a hypertensive crisis.

○ **What hypertensive medications classically cause withdrawal hypertension and, therefore, should not be stopped prior to surgery?**

Beta-blockers and clonidine.

○ **When is the risk of rebound hypertension from propranolol withdrawal the greatest?**

4 to 7 days after the drug is discontinued.

○ **Of Goldman's risk factors, which has been shown to be the most significant?**

Congestive heart failure (CHF).

○   **How does diabetic nephrosclerosis result in rapid renal failure?**

As each nephron is lost, the remaining glomeruli are exposed to more and more hyperfiltration.

○   **What is the appropriate preoperative work-up for a young patient with frequent premature ventricular contractions (PVCs)?**

An ECG, holter monitor and a cardiac stress test.

○   **When should a patient quit smoking to have the greatest decrease in perioperative pulmonary complications?**

8 weeks before the planned procedure.

○   **What percentage of patients requiring amputation of the lower extremity are diabetic?**

60%.

○   **Which artery is usually the first to succumb to large vessel atherosclerosis in the diabetic patient?**

The anterior tibial artery.

○   **What is the accepted stress dose of corticosteroids for patients undergoing major procedures?**

Hydrocortisone, 100 mg, the night before the procedure with repeat administration every 8 hours until the stress has passed.

○   **What is the advantage of administering a blood transfusion the day before a planned procedure as opposed to the day of the surgery?**

Transfused blood is low in 2,3-DPG (less oxygen delivery). In addition, there may be fewer problems with volume shifts and fluid overload.

○   **What is the incidence of thrombocytopenia in HIV+ patients and those with AIDS?**

13 and 43%, respectively.

○   **When should oral hypoglycemics be discontinued prior to surgery?**

24 hours.

○   **How is the creatinine level affected by age?**

As age increases, muscle mass declines. Creatinine production is directly linked to muscle mass. However, since glomerular filtration rate (GFR) declines with age, creatinine remains about the same. Thus, identical creatinine levels may reflect vastly different GFRs.

○   **What cardiac problems almost always mandate a delay of elective surgery?**

Recent myocardial infarction (MI), unstable or severe angina, decompensated CHF, high-grade atrioventricular block, symptomatic ventricular arrhythmias and severe valvular disease.

○   **What factors are important in predicting perioperative morbidity and mortality in patients with cirrhosis?**

Serum bilirubin and albumin, ascitis, encephalopathy and nutritional status.

❍ **T/F: Outpatient surgery is reserved for ASA class I and II patients.**

False.

❍ **At what serum potassium level should elective surgical procedures be aborted?**

Over 6 mEq/l or below 3 mEq/l.

❍ **When should warfarin therapy be discontinued prior to surgery?**

96 to 115 hours (4 doses).

❍ **What factors increase the risk of postoperative pulmonary embolism (PE)?**

Age greater than 40 years, history of lower extremity venous disease, malignancy, CHF, trauma and paraplegia.

❍ **What electrolyte abnormality is a risk factor for precipitating digitalis toxicity?**

Hypokalemia.

❍ **What are the indications for preoperative hemoglobin testing?**

Anticipated major blood loss, pregnancy, suspicion of anemia, renal insufficiency, malignant disease, recent immigration, institutionalized patients over 75 years of age, DM and cardiac disease.

❍ **What are the indications for preoperative determination of serum potassium levels?**

Diuretic therapy, diarrhea, DM, renal disease, inability to provide a history and patients older than 60 years of age.

❍ **What are the indications for preoperative liver function testing?**

Known liver disease, history of hepatitis and malignant disease.

❍ **What are the advantages of a thallium stress test over an exercise stress test?**

The thallium stress test can better identify the location and extent of myocardial ischemia.

❍ **Children may have unlimited clear liquids up to how many hours prior to scheduled anesthetic induction?**

2 to 3 hours.

❍ **T/F: Individuals who take clear liquids close to their time of surgery are at greater risk of aspiration than those who remain NPO.**

False.

❍ **In emergency surgery following trauma, what organisms are most likely to cause serious sepsis?**

Gram-negative bacteria.

❍ **What pre-existing conditions can alter host resistance to infection?**

DM, endogenous or exogenous steroids and NSAIDs.

❍ **How is vitamin A associated with natural immunity?**

It is a component of a complete inflammatory reaction and an adjuvant in the development of specific antibodies.

O   **T/F: The operating room team is the primary source of perioperative infection.**

False.

O   **Wound infections that occur in clean operations are most commonly caused by what organisms?**

Staphylococci.

O   **What is considered a clean-contaminated wound?**

One in which the alimentary, respiratory or genitourinary tracts are entered under controlled conditions and without unusual contamination, minor break in technique or mechanical drainage.

O   **How do hematomas increase the risk of infection?**

They prevent fibroblast migration and capillary formation.

O   **What is the incidence of a wound infection in wounds that contain greater than 100,000 bacteria/gram of tissue?**

50 to 100%.

O   *What is the source of fever in atelectasis?*

Alveolar Macrophages.

O   **When should sutures be removed from areas of good blood supply (i.e., face and neck)?**

Within 4 or 5 days.

O   **T/F: Patients with biliary obstruction should receive vitamin K prior to surgery.**

True.

O   **What is the risk of perioperative MI in patients undergoing surgery within 3 to 6 months of an MI?**

16%.

O   **What drug decreases the incidence of perioperative mortality in patients with idiopathic hypertrophic subaortic stenosis (IHSS)?**

Beta-blockers.

O   *After patient undergoes general anesthesia, his temperature increases to 104 and his end tidal CO2 increases. He develops diffuse muscle rigidity. What causes this condition and what are its treatments?*

Malignant hyperthermia is caused by Ca release from the Sarcoplasmic reticulum.
It is best treated with supportive care, stopping offending agent and Dantrolene

O   **What parameter best correlates with the need for postoperative ventilatory support?**

Arterial CO2.

O   **What is the acceptable level of preoperative factor VIII in patients with hemophilia A?**

Greater than 80% of normal.

❍ ***What organ detects low Na/Cl and produces renin? And what will renin do?***
Renin- produced in macula densa of kidney will convert angiotensinogen to Angiotensin I.

❍ **What is the appropriate tetanus prophylaxis for a patient with a tetanus-prone wound, who has not been previously immunized?**

0.5 ml absorbed toxoid and 250 units of human tetanus immune globulin.

❍ ***What is the difference between sensitivity and specificity?***

Sensitivity= ability to detect a disease.. tp/tp+fn.. A sensitive test has low FN. Positive in disease.
Specificity=ability to say that no disease is present. tn/tn+fp..specific test has low FP. Negative in health.

❍ **What type of suture causes the least amount of tension on wound edges?**

Interrupted perpendicular sutures.

❍ **What is the most common site of perforation of the surgeon's glove during surgery?**

The nondominant index finger.

❍ ***What are type I and type II statistical error?***

Type I- is when you reject the Null hypothysis and the hypothysis is true.
Type II is when you falsely accept the null hypothesis.
Type III is when conclusions are not supported by the data.

❍ **What is the prophylactic antibiotic of choice prior to appendectomy?**

Cefotetan or cefoxitin.

❍ ***What are prevalence and incidence?***

Prevalance is the # of people having the disease in a population.
Incidence is the # of newly diagnosed cases in a population in a certain time.

❍ **What is the primary indication for a closed-suction drain?**

To establish a path of least resistance to the outside.

❍ **T/F: Closure with skin staples causes less necrosis than suturing methods.**

True.

❍ **In what procedures should prophylactic antibiotics be given?**

Most alimentary tract operations, cesarean sections, hysterectomies, selected biliary tract operations and procedures associated with life-threatening consequences should infection occur (e.g., neuorosurgery, cardiovascular procedures and those involving implantable devices).

❍ ***What is needed for conversion to angiotensin II?***

The lung produces A.C.E. This will convert AngiotensinI to Angiotensin II.
Angiotensin II increases Aldosterone release and directly induces vasoconstriction.
Aldosterone enhances renal absorbtion of Na and secretion of K+ & H+ in the urine.

❍   **When are prophylactic antibiotics given during a cesarean section?**

After the umbilical cord is clamped.

❍   **T/F: Cold knife dissection is associated with an increased susceptibility to infection compared to cutting cautery dissection.**

False.

❍   *What is the primary cause of renal ostodystrophy?*

Increase secretion of PTH. Secondary to renal loss of Ca and retention of PO4. There is also a decrease in Vit D 1-hydroxylation in the kidney causing decreased GI absorption of calcium.

❍   **What is the best type of drain for an established enteric fistula?**

A sump drain.

❍   **Hexachlorophene is effective against what organisms?**

Gram-positive bacteria.

❍   **What is the first muscle to return to function after paralytics?**

Diaphragm.

WOUND HEALING AND NUTRITION PEARLS

Oh powerful bacillus, with wonder how you fill us. . .
William T. Helmuth

○ **What is the mechanism of reperfusion injury?**

Production of superoxide and hydroxyl free radicals.

○ *What are the primary nutrition sources for the colon and small bowel?*

Colon- short chain fatty acids; Small Bowel- glutamine.

○ **What is the major disadvantage of delivering TPN through a peripheral vein?**

Limited caloric delivery.

○ **What are the characteristics of the early anabolic (corticoid withdrawal) phase after extensive injury or trauma?**

It follows the catabolic phase within 3 to 8 days and lasts for approximately 2 days. It is characterized by a sharp decline in nitrogen excretion and restoration of appropriate nitrogen balance.

○ *What vitamin reverses the effect of steroids on wound healing?*

Vitamin A

○ **During the inflammatory phase of wound healing, what chemotactic factors attract neutrophils to the wound?**

Complement component C5a and platelet derived growth factor (PDGF).

○ **When can feedings be started after placement of a jejunostomy tube?**

In 12 to 18 hours.

○ *How many Kcal/g does Carbs/proteing/fat contain?*

Carbs- 3.4
Protein- 4
Fat- 9

○ **What is the single best measure of nutritional status?**

Serum albumin level.

○ *What is the order of Cells to a wound?*

Platelets---pmn's---macrophages---fibroblasts.

○ *Contraction is mediated by what cells?*

Myofibroblasts.

○ **Where is Vitamin D made and where is it activated?**

Made in the skin and goes to liver for 25-0H then kidney for 1-OH where it becomes activated.

○ **When does the maturation phase of a normally healing wound occur?**

About 3 weeks after injury.

○ **What is the ratio of Type I to Type III collagen in normal skin?**

8:1.

○ **How does PTH effect gut absorbtion of Ca?**

PTH potentiates vitamin D hydroxylation in the kidney (1-0H). This activated vitamin D augments intestinal Ca absorbtion.

○ **T/F: Urinary nitrogen excretion is proportional to resting energy expenditure (REE).**

True.

○ **What is the function of transforming growth factor-beta (TGF-beta)?**

It stimulates growth of fibroblasts and inhibits growth of epithelial cells.

○ **Where are branched chain amino acids metabolized?**

Muscle.

○ **T/F: Compared to enteral feedings, administration of TPN is associated with an increased incidence of mucosal bacterial translocation.**

True.

○ *What are the products of platelet degranulation?*

TGF-beta and platelet derived growth factor (PDGF).

○ **What are the characteristics of kwashiorkor (acute visceral protein depletion)?**

Edema, variable weight and hypoalbuminemia.

○ **What is the primary cell regulating collagen synthesis?**

The macrophage.

○ *Match the following vitamin deficiency with the clinical presentation*

1. Zinc	a. Decrease in Vit C stores
2. Phosphate	b. anemia, neutropenia

3. *Copper*   *c. dermatitis, hair loss, vision changes*

4. *Lineoleic acid*   *d. hyperglycemia, neuropathy*

5. *Vit A*   *e. perioral rash, hair loss, poor healing,*

6. *Chromium*   *f. weakness, encephalopathy*

1. e   2. f   3. b   4. c   5. a   6. d

○   **Which post-surgical or post-treatment patients would benefit from TPN?**

Generally, patients with massive small bowel resection, severe radiation enteritis, those on high-dose chemotherapy regimens or with a catabolic status lasting 5 to 7 days and those with enterocutaneous fistulas.

○   **What cell secretes pro-alpha collagen chains?**

The fibroblast.

○   **Once glycogen stores are depleted, what is the secondary energy source in the body?**

Protein.

○   **How can the body adjust to prevent protein breakdown?**

By breaking down fatty acids to ketone bodies.

○   **T/F When one re-opens a week old surgical incision the wound will heal slower than an incision in a virgin area?**

False. The matrix of wound healing cells is already laid down, so healing is faster

○   *What is the dominant cell type during the inflammatory phase of wound healing?*

The macrophage.

○   **What peripheral factors contribute to starvation in cancer patients?**

Anorexia, loss of taste and complications from antineoplastic therapies. Mechanical factors related to intake or absorption rarely play a major role.

○   *During prolonged starvation what fuel does the brain use?*

Ketones.

○   **What is the best measurement of marginal malnutrition?**

Retinal-binding prealbumin.

○   **T/F: TPN increases the spontaneous closure of intestinal fistulas.**

True.

○   **T/F: TGF-beta stimulates endothelial cell proliferation.**

False. It inhibits it.

❍ **How much weight loss is clinically significant?**

As a rule, any weight loss exceeding 10% may be significant.

❍ **What serum albumin level is associated with malnutrition?**

Less than 3g/dl.

❍ **T/F: Epithelialization is more rapid under moist conditions than dry conditions.**

True.

❍ **T/F: Large doses of vitamin E enhance wound healing.**

False.

❍ **What serum protein concentration is associated with malnutrition?**

Less than 6 g/dl.

❍ *What electrolyte should be inspected if difficulty correcting pts low Ca?*

Magnesium.

❍ **Where is Vitamin D made and where is it activated?**

Made in the skin and goes to liver for 25-0H then kidney for 1-OH where it becomes activated.

❍ *What metabolic complication occurs when excessive amounts of glucose are infused with the TPN solution?*

Carbon dioxide retention.

❍ *What preoperative laboratory abnormality is most predictive of morbidity and mortality?*

Low serum albumin.

❍ **What is the main difference between a keloid and a hypertrophic scar?**

Keloids extend beyond the boundary of the original tissue injury, hypertrophic scars do not.

❍ **What is the most likely cause of diarrhea in a patient receiving an elemental diet?**

The high osmolarity of the TPN.

❍ **What hormone normally regulates protein synthesis and breakdown?**

Insulin.

❍ *Which amino acid is a key fuel for rapidly dividing cells, including cancer cells?*

Glutamine.

❍ **Which serum proteins can be used to assess short-term nutritional status?**

Transferrin (half-life of 8 to 9 days), prealbumin (half-life of 2 days) and retinal-binding globulin (half-life of 12 hours).

❍ **What factors can influence prealbumin levels?**

Cirrhosis of the liver and hepatitis can reduce prealbumin levels. Renal disease can increase prealbumin levels.

❍ **What is the function of epidermal growth factor (EGF)?**
It stimulates DNA synthesis and cell division in a variety of cells, including fibroblasts, keratinocytes and endothelial cells.

❍ **T/F: Epithelialization produces a watertight seal within 48 hours.**

True.

❍ **How many days of TPN are required to see a measurable response?**

At least 7 to 14 days.

❍ **How is anemia best corrected in patients on TPN?**

Transfusion. In patients who will not accept blood, high dose intravenous iron therapy can be used.

❍ *What TPN additive exerts trophic effects on intestinal mucosa and diminishes bacterial translocation across the gut?*

Glutamine.

❍ **How are maintenance fluids adjusted for febrile patients?**

They are increased by 10 ml/kg for each degree Fahrenheit over 101°.

❍ **T/F: The use of TPN is associated with an increased risk of multiple organ failure (MOF).**

True.

❍ **When should scar revision take place?**

Not for at least 1 year after injury.

❍ **What cells produce GM-CSF?**

Activated T lymphocytes.

❍ **How is the basal metabolic rate (BMR) calculated?**

The modified Harris-Benedict formula is calculated as follows: BMR (kcal/d) = 666 + (9.6 x weight [kg]) + (1.7 x height [cm]) - (4.7 x age [yrs]).

❍ *What is the predominant type of collagen in scar tissue?*

Type I.

❍ *What cells cause contraction of wound edges?*

Myofibroblasts.

❍ **T/F: During starvation, administration of at least 100 gm of glucose exerts a protein-sparing effect mediated by release of endogenous insulin.**

True.

O   **What is the caloric content of 1g of glucose?**

3.4 kcal.

O   **What is the function of laminin?**
It facilitates epithelial cell anchoring.

O   **What fraction of daily protein need can be expected from dietary sources?**

25%.

O   **When can you expect to see a deficiency in essential fatty acids in a fasting patient?**

4 to 6 weeks.

O   **Should TPN be tapered in normoglycemic patients who become hyperglycemic after institution of TPN?**

No. It is important to replete the caloric and fluid needs of the patient. Insulin should be added to TPN to control glucose levels.

O   **What is the role of glutamine in TPN and enteral solutions?**

Glutamine is a nonessential amino acid that carries ammonia. At times of stress, it may become an essential amino acid. There is some evidence to suggest that the addition of glutamine in TPN or enteral formulations may increase nitrogen balance.

O   **If a central line used for TPN becomes clotted, must it be removed?**

It may be possible to save the line by instilling urokinase.

O   **What are the characteristics of linoleic acid deficiency?**

Dermatitis, hair loss, paresthesias and blurred vision.

O   **What is the advantage of cyclic TPN?**

Cyclic TPN can be given over a short period, for example at night, which allows the patient to pursue more normal activities during the day when the TPN is not running.

O   **What percentage of critically ill and injured patients are catabolic or hypermetabolic?**

Nearly 100%.

O   **T/F: Immunocompetence and vital organ function are dependent upon nutritional support.**

True. Both are secondary goals of nutritional support.

O   **With the onset of critical illness, what factors are thought to raise REE and protein turnover?**

Catecholamines and cortisol.

O   **How does the insulin resistance associated with critical illness affect substrate use?**

Insulin resistance decreases the peripheral use of glucose and increases proteolysis.

❍   **What are the serum half-lives of albumin and prealbumin?**

Approximately 20 days and 2 to 3 days, respectively.

❍   **What two methods are frequently relied upon to assess nutritional status in critically ill patients?**

Indirect calorimetry and nitrogen balance.

❍   **What is the equation for nitrogen balance?**

Nitrogen Balance = (Nitrogen intake) - (Nitrogen loss)
                 = (Protein [g] / 6.25) - (Urine Urea Nitrogen / 0.8) + 3.

❍   **How much protein is required for a balanced diet in a healthy adult?**

Approximately 0.6 g/kg ideal body weight per day.

❍   *What is the most common severe complication of enteral nutrition?*

Aspiration.

❍   **What is the recommended starting point for protein replacement in hypermetabolic critically ill patients?**

1.5 to 2.5 g/kg ideal body weight per day.

❍   **T/F: Lipid emulsions are useful in patients needing volume restriction or demonstrating carbohydrate intolerance.**

True. Lipids are calorie-dense compared to dextrose solutions.

❍   **What minimum percentage of total calories should be supplied as lipid to prevent fatty acid deficiency?**

5%.

❍   **How long does it take nonstressed patients receiving lipid-free TPN to demonstrate evidence of essential fatty acid deficiency?**

Within 4 weeks (hypermetabolic patients may do so within 10 days).

❍   **What cells produce interferon (IFN)?**

Lymphocytes and fibroblasts.

❍   **When does tensile strength correlate with total collagen content?**

For about the first 3 weeks of wound healing.

❍   *What clinical symptoms are seen with hypophosphatemia brought on by refeeding a malnourished patient?*

Respiratory insufficiency, muscle weakness, & congestive heart failure.

❍   *What is the main energy source of enterocytes?*

Glutamine.

○   **Besides as an energy source, what role does glutamine play in the gut?**

It is thought to be important in maintaining intestinal structure and function.

○   **Arginine, a semi-essential amino acid, is considered to be vital to what body system?**

The immune system.

○   *T/F: The most common source for pyogenic liver abscess is cholecystitis.*
False, a source is most often not identified.

○   **When should nutritional support be started?**

When a hypermetabolic state (e.g., trauma and sepsis), underlying malnutrition or an expected delay in resuming an oral diet is recognized.

○   **What is the most common metabolic complication of TPN administration in adults?**

Hepatic steatosis (almost always associated with glucose overload).

○   *Sepsis in burn patients is most likely secondary to what source?*

Transmucosal GI bacterial transmission.

○   **What drugs inhibit wound contraction?**

Colchicine, thiphenamil and vinblastine.

○   *T/F: Early initiation of enteral feedings decreases septic complications in trauma patients compared to early parenteral nutrition?*

True.

○   **What are the characteristics of phosphate deficiency?**

Respiratory Weakness, encephalopathy and paresthesias.

○   **T/F: Preoperative nutritional support for malnourished patients has been shown to be effective at reducing postoperative morbidity.**

True. However, it is only effective for patients with severe malnutrition.

○   **In which patients is parenteral nutritional support indicated?**

When enteral access is unobtainable, enteral feeding contraindicated or when the level of enteral nutrition fails to meet requirements.

○   **In which patients is intravenous nutritional support unlikely to be of benefit?**

Patients expected to start oral intake in 5 to 7 days and those with mild injuries.

○   **T/F: Underfeeding can result in difficulty in weaning a patient from mechanical ventilation.**

True. Malnutrition can cause respiratory muscle weakness and ventilator dependence.

○   *What does a respiratory quotient (RQ) less than 0.7 indicate?*

Use of ketones as the source of fuel(Lipolysis).

○   **T/F: TGF-beta enhances angiogenesis.**

True.

○   **T/F: Patients with renal insufficiency should have their protein intake restricted.**

False. Protein restriction is usually only necessary in patients who are unable to undergo dialysis.

○   **What are the advantages of enteral nutrition when compared to parenteral nutrition?**
Enteral nutrition is more physiologic, has a trophic effect on gastrointestinal cells, avoids the need for a central venous catheter, is associated with fewer complications and costs less.

○   **What does indirect calorimetry measure?**

Gas exchange at steady-state. Measured values include inspired and expired oxygen fractions, inspired and expired carbon dioxide fractions and minute ventilation. Oxygen consumption and carbon dioxide production are calculated using these measurements.

○   ***Burn wound infection is best documented by what means?***

Tissue biopsy.

○   **A previously healthy 20 year old female is injured in a motor vehicle accident (MVA). The day following admission her serum albumin is noted to be 2.8 g/dl. Why is her serum albumin low?**

Hypoalbuminemia in acute illness is due to the acute phase protein response, hemodilution from resuscitation and transcapillary escape of albumin to the interstitium.

○   **What happens to nitrogen reserves after trauma?**

They are mobilized due to accelerated protein catabolism.

○   **TGF-beta acts as a chemotactic agent for what cells?**

Fibroblasts, monocytes and macrophages.

○   ***What laboratory abnormality is highly predictive of an increased rate of perioperative morbidity and mortality?***

Low serum albumin.

○   **A critically ill patient's intravenous access is via a peripherally inserted central catheter. Can solutions with an osmolarity of greater than 900 mOsm be infused through it?**

Yes. Although the insertion site is peripheral, the catheter tip is in a central vein and, thus, there is no osmolarity restriction.

○   **What minimum length of small bowel is required for enteral absorption of nutrients?**

100 cm.

○   **What is the essential fatty acid requirement of an adult?**

2 to 4% of calories as linoleic acid.

❍   *What are the clinical manifestations of hypomagnesemia?*

Anorexia, tachyarrythmias, nausea, vomiting, lethargy, weakness, positive Trousseau's and Chvostek's sign, tremor and muscle fasciculations.

❍   **Which type of collagen is a crucial component of the basement membrane?**

Type IV.

❍   **What percentage of most lipid emulsions are essential fatty acids?**

50 to 75%.

❍   **When fat emulsions are administered, which patients should have monitoring of serum triglyceride levels?**

Patients with hyperlipidemias, acute pancreatitis, pulmonary insufficiency, hepatic failure and sepsis.

❍   **At what level of serum triglycerides should fat and glucose administration be decreased?**

If it exceeds 500 mg/dl.

❍   **What is the most common organism associated with catheter sepsis from long-term TPN?**

Staphylococcus aureus.

❍   **When ordering TPN, the concentrations of what electrolytes must be monitored to prevent precipitation?**

Calcium and phosphate.

❍   *What is the leading cause of hospital acquired bactermia?*

Central line infection.

❍   **What is the indication for increasing the acetate concentration in TPN solutions?**

Metabolic acidosis, usually non-anion gap acidosis in which bicarbonate loss is the cause of the acidosis.

❍   **What nutritional deficiency should be considered if a patient has unexplained lactic acidosis?**

Thiamin.

❍   *What is the respiratory quotient for carb/prot/fat.*

Pure glycolysis - 1
Protein- .8
Lipolysis - .7
Lipogenesis RQ > 1

❍   *What is one of the earliest metabolic signs of systemic sepsis?*

Glucose intolerance.

❍   **A patient on TPN has severe diarrhea. What trace element may need to be supplemented?**

Zinc.

❍ **What is the effect of parenteral lipid administration on cellular immunity?**

It causes reticuloendothelial dysfunction and immune suppression.

❍ **T/F: Pulse oximeters detect carboxyhemoglobin with a decreased O2 saturation reading.**

False, the 02 sat levels remain normal.

❍ **An order is placed for multi-trace elements as MTE-5. What 5 trace elements are included?**

Zinc, copper, chromium, manganese and selenium.

❍ **An order is placed for multivitamins as MVI-12. What vitamin is excluded and must be added separately to TPN solutions?**
Vitamin K.

❍ *What vitamin deficiency can be caused by gastric or ileal resection?*

Vitamin B12.

❍ **The stress of illness is associated with a decrease in serum iron and zinc. What happens to these trace elements?**

They are sequestered in tissue, especially in the liver. There are also increased zinc losses in the urine.

❍ **How is first-pass metabolism affected by TPN?**

First-pass metabolism is not preserved during TPN administration.

❍ *The most effective way to reduce ventillator associated pneumonia is?*

Regular airway suctioning with closed catheters.

❍ **What is the goal for calculated nitrogen balance in a critically ill patient?**

Positive 2 to 6 grams of nitrogen per day.

❍ **Why is the use of transferrin as a marker of visceral protein stores limited?**

Transferrin levels may be affected by factors other than nutritional status, such as iron deficiency anemia, liver disorders and neoplastic diseases.

❍ *What are the untoward effects of overfeeding in a critically ill patient?*

Increased carbon dioxide production, increased oxygen consumption, fluid overload, hepatic steatosis and hyperglycemia.

❍ **What are the indications for tube feeding via the jejunal route?**

Comatose patients, patients without a laryngeal reflex and those in whom nasoesophageal, nasogastric or nasojejunostomy tubes cannot be placed.

❍ **T/F: Thromboxane A2 synthesis is increased during vascular injury and arteriosclerosis with endothelial denudation.**

True.

○   **T/F: Tensile strength will reach original skin strength in 6 months.**

False. Original strength is never regained.

○   **What are the two most common causes of hyperphosphatemia?**

Acute and chronic renal failure.

○   **What is the effect of prostacyclin on vascular smooth muscle tone?**

It is inhibitory.

○   **What is the role of chromium in human metabolism?**

Chromium promotes insulin action in peripheral tissues.

○   **Which hormones are influenced by the body's response to injury?**

Catecholamines, aldosterone, antidiuretic hormone, cortisol and growth hormone.

○   **T/F: In the first 12 to 24 hours after major trauma, blood glucose and insulin levels are expected to be high.**

False. During the initial ebb phase, blood glucose is elevated with low insulin levels. After 24 hours the hypermetabolic phase predominates with elevated glucose and insulin.

ANESTHESIA PEARLS

Mr. Anesthetist, if the patient can keep awake, surely you can.
Wilfred Trotter

O   *What is the risk of halothane anesthesia?*

Hepatitis with Fever, eosinophilia and jaundice.

O   **How do volatile anesthetics affect respiratory muscle function?**

They depress synaptic transmission, preferentially affecting the intercostal muscles.

O   **What percentage of anesthetics induce atelectasis at 1 hour post-surgery? At 24 hours post-surgery?**

90% at one hour, 50% at 24 hours.

O   **What antiemetic agent increases gastric motility?**

Reglan (metoclopromide).

O   **How often is phrenic nerve paralysis found after cardiac surgery?**

In fewer than 10% of patients.

O   *What conscious sedation agent is often used with children that increases cardiac work, secretions and BP, and is not associated with respiratory depression?*

Ketamine.

O   **What muscle is typically the first to recover from paralytic therapy ?**

The diaphragm.

O   **What variables are associated with severe atelectasis following cardiac surgery?**

The number of saphenous vein grafts, the use of internal mammary artery grafts, the length of cardiac by-pass time and whether or not the pleural space was entered.

O   **What is the classic mechanism of phrenic nerve injury during cardiac surgery?**

Phrenic nerve frostbite from the cardioplegia solution. The phrenic nerve can also be mechanically injured in the dissection of the internal mammary artery because of its anatomic proximity.

O   **What proposed mechanism of atelectasis is unique to cardiac surgery?**

Cardioplegia solution finding its way into the pulmonary circulation. It is postulated that the high potassium chloride content of the solution damages pulmonary endothelial cells.

O   **How can the incidence of post-cardiac surgery atelectasis be decreased?**

The use of careful technique in mobilizing the internal mammary artery, using a pericardial insulating pad, avoiding entry into the pleural space and recovery of as much cardioplegia solution as possible before it enters the pulmonary circulation.

O   **What is the death rate from anesthesia in patients with an ASA class I or II?**

1 in 200,000.

O   *T/F: Clindamycin prolongs the effect of nondepolarizing muscle relaxants.*

True.

O   **What is the inheritance pattern and incidence of pseudocholinesterase deficiency?**

Autosomal recessive with an incidence of about 1 in 3000.

O   **How is the allowable blood loss (ABL) for a patient calculated?**

In adults, estimated blood volume (EBV) is 60 to 70 cc/kg. ABL = EBV x (Hg [initial] - Hg [final] / Hg [initial]).

O   **In patients planned for a coronary artery bypass graft (CABG), what is the incidence of carotid disease?**

Up to 38%.

O   **How does renal failure affect the cardiac status of a patient?**

These patients are often plagued by hypertension, volume overload, anemia, accelerated atherosclerosis and electrolyte abnormalities.

O   **What med is associated with decrease splanchnic blood flow?**

Vasopressin- therefore used in gi bleeds.

O   **T/F: Beta-blocker eye drops can cause bronchoconstriction in patients under anesthesia.**

True.

O   **What patients may have detrimental side effects from succinylcholine?**

Those with closed-angle glaucoma, space-occupying intracranial lesions and those with severe crush injuries of the lower extremity.

O   **Patients requiring an emergency tracheostomy for an obstructed airway may develop what postoperative pulmonary complication?**

Pulmonary edema.

O   *What is the treatment for malignant hyperthermia?*

Cessation of anesthesia, administration of dantrolene and general supportive measures.

O   *Which local anesthetics are amide compounds?*

Lidocaine and bupivocaine.

O   **What is the FEV1 below which a patient may not have general anesthesia?**

There is no absolute cutoff. There are reports of patients having general anesthesia safely with an FEV1 of around 450 ml.

O   *Why do we wrap the Sodium Nitroprusside bottle in aluminum foil?*

To avoid the breakdown products of SN. Most notably CYANIDE, light enhances the formation of CN.

O   **What is the benefit of preoperative pulmonary prophylactic measures in patients with COPD?**

Decreased pulmonary complications.

O   **Should surgery be delayed in an asthmatic patient who is wheezing?**

If the patient does not always wheeze and their pulmonary status can be improved, then delaying the surgery would seem reasonable. There are some asthmatic patients who, in spite of the appropriate medications, always wheeze. There may be no benefit to delaying surgery in these patients.

O   **What makes midazolam particularly useful in the outpatient setting?**

It has a relatively short onset of action and an elimination half-life of 2 to 4 hours.

O   **What role might oral clonidine play in the preoperative period?**

As an alpha-2 adrenergic agonist, it can reduce anesthetic requirements and has been used to provide sedation and anxiolysis while maintaining hemodynamic stability.

O   **Which local anesthetic produces toxicity at the lowest dose?**

Tetracaine.

O   **By what mechanism does pulse oximetry provide accurate measurement of oxygen saturation?**

Pulse oximetry is based on Beer's law, which relates the concentration of a solute in suspension (in this case, hemoglobin) to the intensity of light transmitted through the solution.

O   **What is the definitive clinical test for complete reversal of neuromuscular blockade?**

The ability of the patient to sustain a head lift from the bed for 5 minutes.

O   **What is the standard endocarditis prophylaxis for dental, oral or upper airway procedures in adult patients at risk?**

Amoxicillin, 3.0 gm orally, 1 hour before the procedure and 1.5 gm 6 hours after the initial dose.

O   **What is the cause of most anesthetic-related deaths?**

Human error (50 to 75%).

O   **What are the most common problems associated with adverse anesthetic outcomes?**

Those related to the airway (i.e., inadequate ventilation, unrecognized esophageal intubation and unrecognized disconnection from the ventilator).

O   **How does the presence of an upper respiratory infection (URI) in an infant influence the perioperative risk of respiratory complications?**

Intubation results in edema and a greater reduction in cross-sectional area of the trachea.

O   **What is the best time to administer oral ranitidine for prophylaxis against acid aspiration?**
60 minutes before induction of anesthesia.

O   *What is the single most important factor predicting postoperative cardiac morbidity?*

History of congestive heart failure (CHF).

O   **What PaO2 level does cause a significant change in oxygen saturation begin to occur?**

Less than 80 mm Hg.

O   **What factors increase the risk of perioperative cardiac complications?**

Greater than 5 premature ventricular contractions (PVCs) per minute, withdrawal of beta-blockers and topical nitrates, presence of CHF and known 3-vessel coronary artery disease (CAD).

O   **What is the principal anesthetic technique used in patients with significant pulmonary disease?**

Intubation at a deep level of anesthesia.

O   **What does end-tidal CO2 measurement reflect?**

Metabolism, circulation and ventilation.

O   **What is the mechanism of action of metoclopramide?**

It inhibits dopamine and enhances the release of acetylcholine, resulting in an increased rate of gastric emptying and increased lower esophageal sphincter (LES) tone. It also inhibits the chemoreceptor zone.

O   **What are the extrapyramidal effects of droperidol?**

Acute dystonia, parkinsonism and akathesia.

O   **What is the single most important factor that determines the length of stay after general anesthesia in ambulatory patients?**

Post-anesthesia nausea.

O   **What are the advantages of propofol over volatile agents in pediatric ambulatory patients?**

Decreased postoperative nausea and vomiting and a decreased incidence of airway obstruction.

O   **How does neostigmine decrease postoperative nausea and vomiting?**

It increases LES pressure and counteracts the increased risk of regurgitation of gastric contents after atropine administration (which lowers LES).

O   **What are the advantages oral midazolam over oral ketamine as a premedicant?**

Oral midazolam has a shorter recovery time and lower cost.

O   **What factors should the ideal premedication in children 1 to 6 years of age possess?**

An atraumatic route of administration, rapid and reliable onset, minimal side effects and rapid elimination.

❍   **What is a reliable alternative induction technique in a 5 year old struggling child who refuses the mask and cannot be managed by intravenous induction because of lack of accessible veins?**

A sedating intramuscular injection of ketamine (3 mg/kg).

❍   **What are the most common anesthetic complications seen in the PACU?**

Nausea, vomiting and airway compromise.

❍   **T/F: All local anesthetics are weak bases and produce vasodilation.**

False. Cocaine is the exception.

❍   **After an oral dose of midazolam, when is it appropriate to separate children from their parents?**

Between 10 and 30 minutes.

❍   **What patients are best suited for oral ketamine?**

Severely stressed and mentally handicapped individuals.

❍   **How should the recovery phase of an ambulatory patient differ from that of an inpatient?**

It should be as brief as possible and be associated with minimal postanesthetic sequelae.

❍   **What may result from an intra-arterial injection of thiopental?**

Crystal formation and local norepinephrine release that may culminate in thrombosis and severe ischemia of the extremity.

❍   **What is the treatment for an intra-arterial injection of thiopental?**

Intravascular dilution and perivascular infiltration with local anesthetic, sympathetic block of the extremity and anticoagulation with heparin.

❍   **How does the half-life of flumazenil compare to that of midazolam?**

The half-life of flumazenil is shorter.

❍   **What effect does etomidate have on the cardiovascular and respiratory systems?**

None.

❍   ***What effects of ketamine discourage its use in patients with increased intracranial pressure (ICP)?***

It causes sympathetic nervous system stimulation, with a rise in blood pressure, heart rate and ICP.

❍   **What factors determine cerebral blood flow?**

Arterial CO_2 and O_2 tension, systemic arterial blood pressure, head position, jugular venous obstruction and positive end-expiratory pressure (PEEP).

❍   **What are the cardiovascular effects of propofol?**

Cardiovascular depression, by a combination of direct myocardial effects and vasodilatation.

❍   **What is the second gas effect of nitrous oxide?**

The ability of nitrous oxide to increase the uptake of other, more potent, inhaled agents.

❍ *What is the most sensitive indicator of a falling cardiac output (CO) during surgery?*

Mixed venous oxygen tension will decrease.

❍ **What anesthetic considerations must be taken into account in a patient with sickle cell disease?**

Adequate hydration and oxygenation. Spinal or local anesthesia should be used whenever possible.

❍ **What are the advantages of nitrous oxide?**

It has a low solubility, is nonflammable, easy to administer and inexpensive.

❍ **Among the currently available potent inhaled anesthethic agents, which ones have a pleasant odor and are not irritating to the airway?**

Halothane and sevoflurane.

❍ **What anesthetic considerations must be taken into account in a patient with ascites?**

Ascites decreases the ventilation-perfusion (V/Q) ratio in the basilar sections of the lung, decreases diaphragmatic excursion, compresses the vena cava and increases the volume of distribution of anesthetic drugs.

❍ **What effect does halothane have on the liver?**

Halothane undergoes significant metabolic degradation, generating compounds that may cause halothane-associated hepatic toxicity.

❍ **What are the cardiovascular effects of isoflurane?**

Myocardial depression, decreased systemic vascular resistance (SVR) and myocardial steal in patients with CAD.

❍ **What patient population might have a decreased amount of pseudocholinesterase?**

Patients taking anticholinesterase medications for glaucoma or myasthenia gravis, chemotherapeutic drugs and patients with a genetically atypical enzyme.

❍ **What are the adverse side effects of succinlycholine?**

Cardiac dysrhythmias, fasciculations, hyperkalemia, myalgia, myoglobinuria, increased pressures (ocular, gastric and cranial), trismus, allergic reactions and it is a trigger for malignant hyperthermia.

❍ **What is the mechanism of action of nondepolarizing neuromuscular blocking agents?**

They combine with nicotinic cholinergic postjunctional receptors. However, they do not activate the receptor or directly block the channel.

❍ **Which neuromuscular blocking agent might be best in an ambulatory patient with significant renal or liver disease?**

Atracurium. It undergoes spontaneous degradation.

❍ *Which inhalational agent is the worst offender in terms of sensitizing the myocardium to catecholamines?*

Halothane.

❍   What are the limits of epinephrine injection when given for hemostasis?

Clinically, epinephrine is limited to 2 mcg/kg with isoflurane. Epinephrine concentrations greater than 1:100,000 increase the risk of ectopy without improving hemostasis.

❍   How is mivacurium metabolized?

By plasma cholinesterase, at a rate approximately 70 to 88% that of succinylcholine. Prolonged recovery has been reported in patients homozygous for atypical pseudocholinesterase enzyme.

❍   *Which nondepolarizing neuromuscular blocking agent might be best in an ambulatory patient who is particularly sensitive to blood pressure changes?*

Vecuronium. It is the only neuromuscular blocking agent essentially devoid of cardiovascular side effects.

❍   Why is regional anesthesia associated with a lower incidence of deep venous thrombosis than general anesthesia?

The maintenance of spontaneous ventilation.

❍   What effect does local infiltration of bupivacaine have on postoperative pain after laparoscopic tubal ligation?

Mesosalpinx infiltration of 0.5% bupivacaine significantly lowers pain intensity and need for postoperative narcotic analgesics.

❍   What regional nerve blocks can be performed to provide postoperative analgesia after inguinal hernia repair in children?

Ilioinguinal and iliohypogastric nerve blocks.

❍   What is an effective alternate analgesic to opioids in a 22 year old healthy female having a laparoscopic tubal ligation?

Preoperative ketolorac.

❍   In terms of duration of action, how does a single dose of fentanyl (1 mcg/kg IV) compare with a single dose of ibuprofen (800 mg PO)?

The therapeutic effects of a single dose of ibuprofen may last more than 4 hours, whereas fentanyl lasts no longer than 2 hours.

❍   What are the advantages of using propofol instead of thiopental for induction and/or maintenance in pediatric patients undergoing ambulatory surgery?

Continuous infusion of propofol is a well-tolerated anesthetic technique in children. The speed and quality of recovery after propofol are superior to that observed after thiopental and/or halothane administration and it is associated with an extremely low incidence of vomiting.

❍   What are the benefits of using sevoflurane over isoflurane in adult ambulatory surgical patients?

Sevoflurane results in faster recovery and decreased side effects.

❍   What are the possible mechanisms for opioid-induced nausea and vomiting?

Delayed gastric emptying, sensitization of the vestibular center and direct action at the chemoreceptor trigger zone.

O   **At what age are infants usually not bothered by separation anxiety?**

Less than 6 months of age.

O   **T/F: A child with congenital heart disease is not a candidate for ambulatory surgery.**

False. A child who has stable congenital heart disease and is being followed by a pediatrician or cardiologist may be an appropriate candidate for ambulatory surgery.

O   **What are the advantages of regional anesthesia?**

It bypasses many of the potential sources of minor or major morbidity associated with general anesthesia.

O   **What is the maximum dose of bupivacaine with epinephrine?**

3 mg/kg.

O   **Which local anesthetic offers the least likelihood of systemic toxicity when performing intravenous regional anesthesia?**

Prilocaine; due to its short plasma half-life.

O   **After performing an axillary block, why might the medial aspect of the upper arm occasionally be spared?**

If it is innervated by the intercostobrachial nerve (T2), which is not part of the brachial plexus. In many individuals, however, this area is primarily innervated by the medial cutaneous nerve of the arm that is part of the brachial plexus and can be anesthetized with an axillary block.

O   **What are the landmarks in performing a midline lumbar spinal block?**

The iliac crest and the L4 and L5 spinal processes (and/or L3 spinous process).

O   *What is the most feared toxicity of ketorlac (toradol)?*

Renal Toxicity.

O   **What indicates a subarachnoid or subdural injection while test-dosing an epidural with local anesthetic?**

The onset of significant anesthesia of more than 2 or 3 segments within 5 minutes of injection.

O   **At what level does the subarachnoid space terminate in children?**

The S2-S3 or S3-S4 space.

O   **What is transient radicular irritation (TRI)?**

Back pain with radiation down one or both buttocks or legs occurring within 24 hours after surgery.

O   *What is the best parameter in predicting successful weaning from mechanical ventillation?*

Rapid Shallow Breathing Index (RR/TV).

O   **What are the possible causes of TRI?**

Specific local anesthetic toxicity, needle trauma, neural ischemia and pooling of local anesthetics secondary to small-gauge pencil point needles.

O   *How would you determine a loading dose for a drug to reach an effective plasma concentration quickly?*

The loading dose is equal to the product of the desired plasma concentration and the volume of distribution.

O   **What signs and symptoms are associated with ionic contrast media administration?**

Flushing, tachycardia, nausea, volume contraction, high urine osmolality and nephropathy. True allergic reactions to the iodine may precipitate anaphylaxis requiring urgent treatment.

O   **What effects do magnetic fields have on pacemakers?**

The effects are variable. The magnetic fields may generate an internal electrical circuit that affects the pacemaker microcircuitry resulting in failure of normal output. There is also a possibility that the mode of the pacemaker may be switched (i.e., demand to asynchrony).

CRITICAL CARE, SHOCK, FLUIDS AND ELECTROLYTES PEARLS

Nature heals under the auspices of the medical profession.
Haven Emerson

○ **At normal body temperature, what is the average daily insensible water loss?**

600 to 900 ml/day or 8 to 12 ml/kg/day.

○ *What are the consequences of exceedingly rapid sodium replacement in hyponatremia?*

Central pontine myelinolysis (quadriplegia, dysarthria and dysphasia).

○ **What are the common causes of hyperosmolar hyponatremia?**

Hyperglycemia, mannitol and radiologic contrast.

○ *Patients with asymptomatic hyponatremia are best treated in what manner?*

Free water restriction.

○ **T/F: Completely occlusive transparent dressings are preferred for central lines.**

False. This type has the highest infection rate.

○ **What type of dressing has the lowest infection rate?**

Gauze and tape.

○ *What is the EKG finding with severe hyperkalemia? And what is the treatment?*

Treat with Ca to stabilize the cardiac membrane. Bicarb and insulin are adjuncts to lower serum K+. Lasix and kayexalate can also be used but they take longer to have an effect.

○ **What is the preferred site for central venous catheterization?**

Controversial. All three major sites (femoral, internal jugular and subclavian) have advantages and disadvantages that must be weighed.

○ **T/F: Femoral vein catheters have the highest infection rates and should not be used routinely.**

False.

○ **What are the componenets of LR and NS?**

LR= NA- 130, K-4, Ca- 2.7, CL- 109 (similar to electrolytes in chem. 7)
NS= Na 154, CL- 154

O   **T/F: Routine changing of central lines over a wire lowers infection rates.**

False.

O   **T/F: Central lines should be flushed with heparin-containing solutions.**

False. Normal saline flushes have the same catheter occlusion incidence as heparin and heparin is occasionally associated with problematic thrombocytopenia.

O   **What is the maximum intravenous potassium administration?**

40 to 60 mEq/hour.

O   **What are the most common causes of SIADH?**

Malignancies, pulmonary disease, CNS disorders and drugs.

O   **How is urine osmolality calculated?**

Urine osmolality = 2 x (urinary sodium + urinary potassium) + urine urea nitrogen / 2.8.

O   **Overly rapid correction of hyponatremia and hypernatremia are associated with which cerbral complications?**

Hyponatremia- Central pontine myelinosis.
Hypernatremia- Cerebral Edema.

O   *What is the diagnostic test of choice to confirm hypoadrenal shock?*

The ACTH stimulation test.

O   **What is the basal production of lactic acid?**

Approximately 1,440 mEq/day.

O   *How is the fractional excretion of sodium (FeNa) calculated?*

FeNa = [(Una / Pna) / (Ucr / Pcr)] x 100%.

O   *What is the major cause of extrarenal potassium depletion?*

Diarrhea.

O   **At what points during insertion and use of pulmonary artery (PA) catheters should the balloon be inflated?**

When it is in the superior vena cava (SVC). It should remain inflated during any forward movement of the catheter and should be deflated prior to any withdrawal. Once in place, the balloon should be inflated only to the minimum volume necessary to obtain a pulmonary capillary wedge pressure (PCWP).

O   **What patient populations are most likely to benefit from the use of the PA catheters?**

Multiple trauma patients, patients with myocardial infarction and shock and those with shock refractory to volume loading. Perioperative management of patients undergoing cardiac or vascular surgery is also an indication.

O   *What is the formula for corrected Ca?*

Calcium +.8 x (4 - albumin).

○ **What is the formula for corrected Na in hyperglycemia?**

(Glucose-100)/100 x 1.6 + Na.

○ **What are the characteristics of dopamine?**

It is a dopaminergic and beta-1 agonist at low doses and an alpha-agonist at higher doses.

○ **What are the major differences between dopamine and dobutamine?**

Dobutamine lacks alpha-1 effects.

○ **How does dopamine promote diuresis?**

Low-dose dopamine (2 to 4 mcg/kg/min) binds to dopaminergic receptors and increases renal blood flow. It also directly inhibits sodium resorption in the proximal tubule. Even at those low doses, beta-adrenergic activation increases cardiac contractility, which also increases renal blood flow.

○ **How do inotropic agents increase myocardial contractility?**

By increasing intracellular calcium concentration and availability.

○ **What pressures can be measured by the PA catheter?**

Systemic vascular resistance (SVR), pulmonary artery pressure (PAP) and PCWP.

○ **What is meant by wedge pressure?**

Left ventricular end diastolic volume (LVEDV), a measure of the preload on the ventricle.

○ **What assumptions are made in using PCWP as a substitute for LVEDV?**

Most importantly, a stable relationship between LVEDP and LVEDV. Also, that the PCWP is equal to the left atrial (LA) pressure, which is equal to the LVEDP.

○ **Do these assumptions hold true in a typical critically ill patient?**

No.

○ **What are the sources of error in these assumptions?**

PCWP can be different from LA pressure and LVEDP due to pulmonary venous resistance, valvular abnormalities, positive pressure ventilation, positive end-expiratory pressure (PEEP), catheter placement in lung zones I or II and abnormal ventricular compliance.

○ **What is the most common cause of acute adrenal insufficiency?**

Withdrawl of chronic administration of exogenous corticosteroids.

○ **What are the gastrointestinal symptoms of hyperkalemia?**

Nausea, vomiting, intermittent intestinal colic and diarrhea.

○ **How does PA diastolic pressure compare to PCWP as a measure of left heart filling pressures?**

Under normal conditions, the PCWP is usually within a few mm Hg of PA diastolic pressure. Conditions common to critical illness make them more disparate.

○   *What is the cause of respiratory acidosis?*
Retention of CO2 and subsequent increased carbonic acid retention.

○   **Where is the majority of intracellular water located?**

In skeletal muscle.

○   *How does PEEP affect PA catheter measurements?*

Some degree of positive thoracic pressure is transmitted to the pulmonary vasculature and, therefore, is measured by the PA catheter. Placement in zone 3 will lessen but not eliminate the effect.

○   **What parameter, measured by PA catheters, correlates with response to fluid challenge?**

Right ventricular end diastolic volume (RVEDV) less than 140 correlates in a positive fashion with increased cardiac output (CO) upon fluid challenge.

○   *What is the relationship of oxygen saturation of venous blood (SvO2) to oxygen delivery (DO2) and oxygen consumption (VO2)?*

SvO2 is a quick way of determining the adequacy of DO2 and VO2. Assuming arterial oxygen saturation (SaO2) of 95 to 100%, the SvO2 should be greater than 70 to 75%. Less than this indicates that the oxygen supply is suboptimal. Unfortunately, in some conditions, such as sepsis, SvO2 will actually be higher than normal, despite inadequate tissue oxygenation.

○   **Respiratory failure is worsened in spinal injuries at or above which nerve root?**

C2.

○   **What is the treatment for TTP?**

Plasmaphoresis (not splenectomy).

○   **What infectious syndromes can lead to ventilatory insufficiency?**

Botulism, tetanus, campylobacter, polio, diphtheria and Guillain Barre' Syndrome.

○   **What is considered a normal Allen test?**

Palmar blush within 7 seconds of ulnar artery release.

○   *What are the typical PA catheter measurements in hypovolemic shock?*

Low CO, high SVR and low PCWP.

○   **T/F: CO2 excretion is directly related to alveolar ventilation.**

True.

○   *Aminoglycosides are effective against what bacteria, and by what mechanism?*

Aerobic gram negative bacilli (including Pseudomonas aeruginosa), enterococci, staphlococci and streptococci. The mechanism is inhibition of ribosome function.

❍   **What risks are associated with the use of aminoglycosides?**

Prolonged neuromuscular blockade, ototoxicity and nephrotoxicity.

❍   *What is the mechanism of bacterial resistance to aminoglycosides?*

Inhibition of active transport of the drug into the bacterial cell.

❍   *A Pt is undergoing a Lap Choly and suddenly after insufflating the abdomen the pts becomes hypotensive with signs of right heart strain on telemetry. What is one immediate treatment?*

*In CO2 air embolus turn pt with left side down and attmet air aspiration with central
Line in RA.*

❍   *Vancomycin is effective against which bacteria and by what mechanism?*

Gram-positive cocci, including methicillin-resistant Staphyloccocus aureus (MRSA), Staphylococcus epidermidis, enterococcus, diptheroids and Clostridium difficile. The mechanism is by cell membrane binding and alteration.

❍   *What is the mechanism of bacterial resistance to vancomycin?*

Altered bacterial cell walls.

❍   **What is Red Man's Syndrome?**

Flushing of the face and neck, pruritis and hypotension associated with rapid infusion of vancomycin and subsequent release of histamine.

❍   **What more recent problem has arisen with the use of vancomycin?**

Development of vancomycin resistant enterococci (VRE).

❍   *Which inherited disorder will always benefit from splenectomy?*

Hereditary shperocytosis.

❍   **What agents are used to treat VRE?**

Chloramphenicol, novobiocin, synercid, teichoplanin, quinolones and doxycycline.

❍   **What are the major intracellular anions?**

Proteins and phosphates.

❍   *What are the feared reactions of Silvadene, sulfamylon and silver nitrate?*

*Silvadene- neutropenia.
Sulfamylon (mafedine acitate) - acidosis.
Silver nitrate- Hyponatremia and hypochloremia.*

❍   **What is the most common cause of hypoxemia?**

Ventilation/perfusion (V/Q) mismatch.

❍   **A burn patient develops a green slime infection on his burns which smells sweet. What is the Organism?**

Pseudomonas.

O   **Which mitral valve abnormalities can lead to large v waves on the pulmonary artery wedge tracing?**

Mitral stenosis and mitral regurgitation. This is due to overfilling of the left atrium.

O   **T/F: Total serum calcium increases by 0.8 mg/dl for every 1 gram/dl increment of serum albumin above a normal value of 4 gm/dl.**

True.

O   **What is the usual cause of decreased lung compliance in patients with acute respiratory failure?**

A decrease in functional residual capacity (FRC).

O   **How do increases in heart rate (HR) alter the systolic and diastolic components of the cardiac cycle?**

As HR increases and cardiac cycle time decreases, systole time remains relatively constant while diastole time decreases, thereby increasing the ratio of systole/diastole.

O   *What is the formula for 02 delivery?*

C.O. x 02 content.

O   **What is the variables determining O2 content?**

Hgb, 02 sat, PaO2.

O   *What percentage of available oxygen is extracted by the heart?*

70%., thus the coronary sinus has the lowest P02 of any vessel in the body.

O   **What is the mortality rate for patients with multiple organ failure (MOF) complicated by acute renal failure?**

50 to 90%.

O   **How much calcium should be administered to a patient receiving rapid blood transfusions?**

0.2 gm for every 500 ml of blood transfused.

O   *What is the acute compensation for metabolic acidosis?*

Respiratory (hyperventilation) alkalosis.

O   *What factors directly affect DO2?*

Hemoglobin concentration, cardiac output and FIO2.

O   **What is the rate limiting factor of DO2 in normal individuals?**

Availability of adenosine diphosphate (ADP).

O   **What is the predominant stimulus for activation of hypoxic pulmonary vasoconstriction?**

Decreased alveolar oxygen tension.

❍ **When does PADP exceed PCWP?**

In patients with tachycardia or pulmonary hypertension associated with acidosis, hypoxia, pulmonary embolism (PE) or pulmonary parenchymal disease.

❍ **What are the most common causes of hypercalcemia?**

Hyperparathyroidism and cancer with bony metastases.

❍ *How does PEEP effect respiratory dynamics?*

It increases FRC and Lung compliance.

❍ *Where Does EDRFarise?*

It is nitric oxide and is released from endothelial cells. NO precursor is Arganine. NO is a smooth muscle relaxing factor and promotes vasodilation.

❍ *What is the mechanism of action of atrial natriuretic peptide (ANP)?*

Sodium overload and retention results in volume overload that distends the atria. The atria then release ANP, which causes an increase in renal vasodilatation and natriuresis.

❍ *What test indicates that the kidney is conserving sodium?*

Low urinary sodium (< 20 mEq/L).

❍ **What is the role of prostaglandins in sodium homeostasis?**

Prostaglandin synthesis is increased in states of absolute effective volume depletion and serves to maintain the glomerular filtration rate (GFR) and the excretion of salt and water. Inhibition of prostaglandin synthesis (e.g., NSAIDs) under these circumstances can lead to a decline in GFR and sodium overload.

❍ *What are the classic signs of hypocalcemia?*

Perioral numbness/tingling, hyperactive deep tendon reflexes, Cvostek's sign and Trousseau's sign.

❍ *By what mechanism does hypovolemia result in metabolic alkalosis?*

The kidney will resorb sodium and excrete hydrogen ions to maintain intravascular volume.

❍ **What hormones regulate potassium balance?**

Insulin, catecholamines and aldosterone.

❍ *How is PEEP useful in the treatment of adult respiratory distress syndrome (ARDS)?*

It increases FRC, increases lung compliance and re-expands alveoli.

❍ **How does acute metabolic acidosis affect serum potassium?**

Serum potassium increases by 0.8 mEq/l for each 0.1 decline in pH. (Organic acidosis does not affect potassium.)

❍ **Hypermagnesemia is most commonly seen in what patients?**

Those with severe renal insufficiency.

O   **How is the effective oncotic pressure of a body compartment determined?**

By the presence of nondiffusable proteins.

O   **What is the most common cause of metabolic acidosis in surgical patients?**

Circulatory failure with subsequent accumulation of lactic acid.

O   **How would you estimate the total body potassium deficit in a patient with a serum potassium of 3 mEq/l?**

A decrease in serum potassium from 4 to 3 mmol/L corresponds to a 100 to 200 mEq decrement in total body potassium. Each additional fall of 1 mEq/L in serum potassium represents an additional deficit of 200 to 400 mEq.

O   **During which phase of the respiratory cycle should pulmonary artery catheter measurements be made?**

At end-expiration.

O   **What is the effect of succinylcholine on plasma potassium?**

Muscle membrane depolarization results in leakage of potassium, producing an average increase of 0.5 to 1.0 mEq/L in serum potassium. However, when succinylcholine depolarizes muscle that has been previously traumatized or denervated, large increases in serum potassium can occur, causing life-threatening arrhythmias and cardiac arrest.

O   **How is the sodium deficit calculated?**

Sodium deficit = (normal sodium - observed sodium) x total body water. Total body water is .6 x wt (kg).

O   **What are the most common causes of increased dead space in critically ill patients?**

Decreased cardiac output, PE, pulmonary hypertension, ARDS and excessive PEEP.

O   *What are the hypertensive, hypokalemic syndromes?*

Primary hyperaldosteronism, secondary hyperaldosteronism and Cushing's syndrome.

O   **What are two relatively specifics findings in PE on chest x-ray?**

Hampton's hump, an area of lung consolidation with a rounded border facing the hilus and Westermark's sign, a dilated pulmonary outflow tract ipsilateral to the emboli, with decreased perfusion distal to the lesion.

O   **What is the neuropathy of critical illness?**

Primary axonal degeneration of motor and sensory fibers.

O   *What is the most reliable measure of glomerular filtration?*

Creatinine clearance.

O   *What is thought to be the common pathophysiologic pathway in the development of ARDS?*

Injury to the alveolar-capillary interface.

O   **Patients on mechanical ventilation develop hypoventilation based on what factors?**

Increased dead space, overdistention of the lungs, air leaks and massive PE.

O   **What is the recommended dose of bicarbonate in the treatment of metabolic acidosis?**

Not greater than 50 ml of a 7.5% solution. Appropriate ventilation is the primary treatment.

O   **What is the diagnostic test of choice for the neuropathy of critical illness?**

EMG.

O   **What is the earliest sign of volume excess in the postoperative period?**

Weight gain.

O   **What are the clinical features associated with hypernatremia?**

Weakness, twitching, lethargy, obtundation, irritability, seizures and cerebral hemorrhage.

O   **How is the free water deficit in a hypernatremic patient calculated?**

Free water deficit = (0.6 x body weight [kg]) x (known sodium concentration - normal sodium concentration).

O   **How is the most effective level of PEEP determined?**

By measurement of effective compliance.

O   ***What are the major criteria for the diagnosis of ARDS?***

Hypoxia refractory to increasing FIO2, decreased pulmonary compliance, decreased FRC, increased dead space ventilation and a diffuse interstitial pattern on chest x-ray with a normal PCWP.

O   **What effect does intrinsic PEEP have on patients receiving mechanical ventilation?**

It increases elastic work and the work to trigger assisted breaths.

O   **T/F: Beta-blockers affect the serum potassium concentration.**

True. They inhibit uptake of potassium by skeletal muscle.

O   **How can the work of breathing with mechanical ventilation, associated with intrinsic PEEP, be reduced?**

Add CPAP, reduce tidal volume, reduce inspiratory time and increase expiratory time.

O   **What is the most common source of gram-negative infections in patients with septic shock?**

The urinary tract.

O   **A 48 year old male in the SICU has a serum sodium of 120 mEq/l and a blood glucose of 480 mg/ml. What is the treatment for the hyponatremia?**

None.

O   **How does pulmonary hypertension contribute to reduced cardiac output?**

Ventricular septum displacement (ventricular interdependence).

O   **What are the characteristics of high-output renal failure?**

Uremia without a period of oliguria and a daily urine output between 1,000 and 1,500 ml.

O   *What are the characteristics of Class II hemorrhagic shock?*

Loss of 15 to 30% of circulating blood volume, tachycardia and a decrease in pulse pressure.

O   **What is the most common cause of volume deficit encountered in surgery?**

Loss of isotonic fluid.

O   **What evidence of barotrauma can be observed on chest x-ray?**

Pneumomediastinum, pneumothorax, pneumopericardium, subcutaneous emphysema and pulmonary interstitial emphysema.

O   **What are the primary determinants of the work of breathing?**

Minute ventilation, lung and chestwall compliance, airway resistance and intrinsic PEEP.

O   *Under what conditions is CO_2 production increased?*

Lipogenesis, fever and hyperthyroidism.

O   **What is the preferred FIO2 for patients with ARDS?**

The lowest that will maintain an oxygen saturation of approximately 90%.

O   **What is the optimum level of PEEP for a patient with ARDS undergoing mechanical ventilation?**

The lowest level that produces the maximum DO2.

O   **How can adequate tidal volume be delivered to a patient undergoing volume cycled mechanical ventilation and whose endotracheal tube cuff is failing to maintain an adequate seal, without changing the tube?**

Increase the mandatory tidal volume.

O   **Which class of hemorrhagic shock is consistent with a drop in systolic blood pressure?**

Class III.

O   **What are the indications for stress ulcer prophylaxis in critically ill patients?**

Mechanical ventilation and coagulopathy.

O   *What is the preferred position for patients suspected of having an air embolism?*

Left lateral decubitus.

O   **What is the hallmark hemodynamic finding of constrictive pericarditis?**

An early diastolic dip and a late diastolic plateau in the RV pressure curve.

❍   **How often is hypotension seen in patients with cardiac tamponade?**

A systolic blood pressure of less than 100 mm Hg is only seen in about 36% of cases.

❍   **What is the diagnosis if clotted blood is discovered during attempted aspiration for pericardial tamponade?**

Either the ventricle was inadvertently entered or the pericardial hemorrhage was massive.

❍   **What is the mortality of patients with acute RV failure due to PE?**

30%.

❍   **How much of the pulmonary vascular bed must be occluded to cause shock in the setting of PE?**

Greater than 60% in patients with no prior cardiopulmonary disease.

❍   **What is the best initial fluid management for a patient with hemorrhagic shock?**

Lactated Ringer's.

❍   **What are the signs of volume overload?**

Distended veins, bounding pulse, functional murmurs, edema and basilar rales.

❍   **What test confirms the diagnosis of diabetes insipidus (DI)?**

Failure of urine osmolality to increase more than 30 mOsm/l in the first hours of complete fluid restriction.

❍   **What are the treatment options for patients with massive PE and acute cor pulmonale?**

Volume resuscitation and vasopressors followed by heparin, thrombolytics or surgical embolectomy.

❍   **Under what circumstances should surgical embolectomy be strongly considered?**

Any hemodynamically unstable patient with documented massive PE and absolute contraindications to thrombolytic therapy.

❍   **What are the most common causes of cardiogenic shock in the setting of an acute MI?**

Greater than 40% loss of LV myocardium, ventricular wall rupture, septal rupture, LV aneurysm and acute mitral regurgitation due to papillary muscle rupture or dysfunction.

❍   **What is the suspected diagnosis if a patient's blood pressure drops significantly with administration of nitroglycerin in the setting of an acute MI?**

Inferior wall MI with RV involvement.

❍   *How does an intraaortic balloon pump (IABP) increase cardiac output?*

It decreases LV afterload and increases coronary perfusion.

❍   **An IABP increases cardiac output by how much?**

10 to 20%.

❍   **What is the treatment of choice for a patient in cardiogenic shock in the setting of an acute MI?**

Angioplasty.

O   **What is the main determinant of the osmolarity of the extracellular fluid space?**

Serum sodium concentration.

O   **What interventions have improved survival of patients with cardiogenic shock in the setting of an acute MI?**

IABP and angioplasty.

O   **How does thrombolytic therapy improve survival in acute MI?**

It decreases the incidence cardiogenic shock.

O   **What complications may occur following massive blood transfusion?**

Electrolyte and acid-base abnormalities, changes in hemoglobin-oxygen affinity, hypothermia, coagulopathy and dysfunction of various organs.

O   **What is the primary extracellular acid-base buffering system?**

The bicarbonate-carbonic acid system.

O   **What percentage of deaths in patients with acute MIs are caused by ventricular wall rupture?**

10 to 15%. Mortality approaches 100%.

O   **What is the first line treatment for a patient in cardiogenic shock due to RV infarction?**

Aggressive volume replacement.

O   *Initial management of a tracheoinnominate fistula should consist of what?*

Hyperinflation of the tracheostomy tube cuff.

O   **What are the prophylactic recommendations for avoiding dilutional coagulopathy in a patient receiving a massive blood transfusion?**

Administration of 1 or 2 units of fresh frozen plasma (FFP) for every 2 to 10 units of transfused blood.

O   **How is the optimal filling pressure determined for a patient in cardiogenic shock?**

By obtaining a bedside Starling curve and plotting PCWP against cardiac output after repeated small volume boluses or diuresis.

O   *What are the characteristics of the systemic inflammatory response syndrome (SIRS)?*

Absence of infection, body temperature greater than 38°C or less than 36°C, tachypnea or hypoventilation, leukocytosis or leukopenia and tachycardia.

O   **What bicarbonate-carbonic acid ratio is associated with a normal pH?**

20:1.

O   *The best method to avoid ventillator induced lung injury in ARDS is?*

Use smaller tidal volumes.

○ **What is the major risk factor associated with development of MOF?**

Sepsis.

○ *What are the major sources of tumor necrosis factor (TNF) following hypoperfusion?*

The liver and gut.

○ **What is the average survival rate for patients with septic shock?**

40 to 60%.

○ **T/F: The circulatory derangements of septic shock precede the metabolic abnormalities.**

False.

○ **How is VO2 calculated?**

V02 = C(a - v)O2 x CO x 10.

○ **What is the normal whole lung V/Q ratio?**

4 liters of ventilation to 5 liters of blood flow.

○ **What is the normal O2UC in a healthy adult?**

25%.

○ **Why has bicarbonate use been de-emphasized?**

Because of its harmful effects, which include hyperosmolarity, alkalemia, hypernatremia, paradoxical CSF acidosis and increased CO_2 production.

○ **What is the treatment of choice for wide complex tachycardia of uncertain etiology?**

Amiodarone or Lidocaine.

○ **In what patients is inverse ratio ventillation most useful?**

Those with non-compliant lungs (ARDS).

○ **A 49 year old male develops tachycardia following successful resuscitation from cardiac arrest. Would you treat this post-resuscitation rhythm?**

If the patient has a pulse and is hemodynamically stable, no treatment may be necessary. If epinephrine is responsible for the tachycardia, it should resolve quickly. Sustained sinus tachycardia should not be allowed to persist, however, as it increases myocardial oxygen consumption.

○ **A patient presents with an inferior wall MI. He is hypotensive with distended neck veins and clear lung fields. What is the most likely diagnosis?**

RV infarct or ischemia.

○ **What is the treatment for a patient with an inferior MI and second-degree block?**

For symptomatic patients, atropine or transcutaneous pacing is appropriate. However, in patients with type II second-degree heart block or third-degree heart block, atropine should be used with caution. Atropine may increase the atrial rate in this group of patients. This, in turn, may increase nodal refractoriness and further slow the ventricular rate.

O   *What is the treatment of choice for hyperkalemia induced cardiac arrhythmia?*

IV Calcium Gluconate.

O   **T/F: In metabolic acidosis and alkalosis, slow compensation occurs via renal mechanisms.**

True.

O   **What special considerations exist when cardiac arrest occurs in a pregnant patient?**

During chest compression, a wedge under the right hip should be used to minimize aortocaval compression. For the pregnant patient who is unconscious due to airway obstruction, chest thrusts are performed rather than abdominal thrusts.

O   **What are the risks of pericardiocentesis?**

Hemothorax, pneumothorax, hemorrhage from myocardial or coronary artery laceration and tamponade from this hemorrhage.

O   *What are the features of SIRS (systemic inflammatiory response syndrome?*

Tachycardia, Fever/Hypothermia, Leukocytosis, Tachypnia.

O   **What is the normal dietary intake of potassium?**

50 to 100 mEq/day.

O   **What medications may be given via the intraosseous route?**

All medications and fluids may be given via this route.

O   **T/F: In a spontaneously breathing patient with acute lung injury, intubation and the application of enriched FIO2 and PEEP, sufficient to recruit collapsed alveolar units, decreases pulmonary vascular resistance.**

True.

O   **What is the effect of myocardial demand on spontaneous ventilation induced by negative swings in intrathoracic pressure?**

It will be increased.

O   **What processes cause the work of breathing to increase markedly in patients with COPD?**

Increased dead space ventilation, decreased respiratory muscle efficiency and increased airway resistance.

O   *A patient has the following pulmonary artery catheter readings: Cardiac index (CI) of 2.0 l/min, CVP of 2 mm Hg, pulmonary artery occlusion pressure (PAOP) of 7 mm Hg and SVR of 1600 dyne/sec/cm2. What is the most consistent diagnosis and what is the appropriate therapy?*

The patient is hypovolemic and would benefit from fluid resuscitation.

❍ *A patient's pulmonary artery catheter readings reveal a CVP of 12 mm Hg, PAOP of 18 mm Hg, CI of 1.7 l/min and SVR of 1650 dyne/sec/cm2. What is the most appropriate treatment?*

Echocardiography and inotropic support. However, this must be judiciously balanced against increasing myocardial oxygen demand. Depending on the patient's condition, an IABP may be lifesaving.

HEAD, NECK AND ENT PEARLS

Nature, time and patience are the three great physicians.
Bulgarian proverb

O   **What is the lymphatic drainage from the middle and posterior third of the tongue?**

To the submandibular and internal jugular nodes.

O   **Where should sutures be placed in repairing full-thickness lacerations of the pinna?**

Through the cartilage.

O   **What is the most common cause of laryngeal stenosis?**

Trauma.

O   *Old women with a dry mouth and foul smelling breath and pain on lateral face 1 cm anterior to ear. She has been diagnosed with parotiditis, what is her treatment?*

Antibiotics, which cover Staph. However drainage required if abscess or not improving.

O   **What effect can CO2 lasers have on the eyes?**

Exposure to a 10,600 nm wavelength produced by the CO2 laser can cause corneal opacification because energy is largely absorbed on the surface of the eye.

O   **T/F: Most carcinomas of the ear are related to excessive sun exposure.**

True.

O   **Where are verrucous carcinomas most commonly found?**

On the inside of the cheek.

O   **Where are most esophageal foreign bodies found?**

Just below the cricopharyngeus muscle.

O   **What is the mechanism of postobstructive pulmonary edema or negative pressure pulmonary edema?**

Forced inspiration against a closed glottis, inducing large negative intrapleural and transpulmonary pressure gradients. This promotes transudation of edema fluid from the pulmonary capillaries into the interstitium.

O   **What is the treatment for edema induced by partial glottic or subglottic airway obstruction?**

Humidified oxygen, adequate hydration and, if necessary, corticosteroids alone or in combination with nebulized racemic epinephrine.

O   **Which organism most commonly causes otitis media in the newborn?**

E. coli.

O   **Which topical anesthetics have been shown to induce methemoglobinemia?**

Prilocaine, benzocaine, lidocaine and procaine.

O   **T/F: Middle ear effusions may cause a conductive hearing loss.**

True.

O   **T/F: Erythroplakia is a premalignant condition?**

True.

O   **T/F: Retinoids can reverse leukoplakia and reduce chance of neck malignancy?**

True.

O   **What is the most common cause of stridor in a newborn?**

Laryngomalacia.

O   **What is the recommended treatment for large carcinomas of the paranasal sinuses?**

Combination surgery, radiation therapy and chemotherapy.

O   **T/F: Glottic carcinomas usually produce symptoms early in the disease process.**

True.

O   **What are the most common problems associated with middle ear surgery?**

Nitrous oxide-induced changes in middle ear pressure, bleeding, facial nerve injury, cervical spine injury, nausea, vomiting and vertigo.

O   **What are the generally accepted indications for tonsillectomy and adenoidectomy (T & A)?**

Airway obstruction, sleep apnea, recurrent tonsil infections, recurrent ear infections, peritonsillar abscess and unilateral tonsillar enlargement.

O   **What is the recommended method for removing impacted cerumen for the external auditory canal?**

3% hydrogen peroxide ear drops.

O   **What genetic syndrome is commonly associated with lymphoid hyperplasia resulting in severe upper airway obstruction?**

Down's syndrome (Trisomy 21).

O   **What are the signs of ongoing bleeding after T & A?**

Frequent swallowing, tachycardia and hypotension.

O   **What is the main determinant of cosmetic outcome in repair of full-thickness lip lacerations?**

Proper apposition of the vermilion border.

❍ **What is the most common malignant salivary tumor?**

Mucoepidermoid Carcinoma.

❍ **What is the most common malignant salivary tumor of the submandibular glands?**

Adenoid Cystic Carcinoma.

❍ **What is the treatment of pleomorphic adenoma?**

Superficial parotidectomy with facial nerve preservation.

❍ **What are the #1 and #2 most common benign salivary tumor?**

#1- pleomorphic adenoma.
#2- Warthin's tumor- 10% are bilateral.

❍ **What is the disadvantage of using PVC, red rubber or silicone endotracheal tubes during laser surgery?**

Each of these tubes can be ignited by the carbon dioxide laser in an environment of 100% oxygen.

❍ **Which part of the airway shows the greatest degree of inflammation in a child with laryngotracheobronchitis (croup)?**

The subglottic region.

❍ **A patient presents with gingival pain and a foul mouth odor. Physical examination reveals fever, lymphadenopathy, bright red gingiva and ulcerated papillae with a gray membrane. What is the most likely diagnosis?**

Acute necrotizing ulcerative gingivitis.

❍ **What is the treatment of choice for the above patient?**

Antibiotics (tetracycline or penicillin) and topical anesthetics.

❍ **What is the most common oral manifestation of AIDS?**

Oropharyngeal thrush.

❍ **What is the most common cause of vertigo in a child?**

Otitis media.

❍ **What complications must be considered in patients with nasal fractures?**

Septal hematoma and cribriform plate fractures.

❍ **What is the treatment for thyroid lymphoma?**

Chemo and radiation therapy.

❍ **What physical exam findings would make posterior epistaxis more likely than anterior epistaxis?**

Inability to see the site of bleeding, blood from both sides of the nose, blood trickling down the oropharynx and inability to control bleeding by direct pressure.

○   **A child with a sinus infection presents with proptosis, a red swollen eyelid and an inferolaterally displaced globe. What is the most likely diagnosis?**

Orbital cellulitis and abscess associated with ethmoid sinusitis.

○   **An ill-appearing patient presents with a fever of 103 °F, bilateral chemosis, 3rd nerve palsy and sinusitis. What is the most likely diagnosis?**

Cavernous sinus thrombosis.

○   **Retropharyngeal abscess is most common in what age group?**

6 months to 3 years (retropharyngeal lymph nodes regress in size after the age of three).

○   **What are the most common types of malignant neoplasms of the nasopharynx in adults?**

Squamous cell carcinoma and its variant, lymphoepithelioma.

○   **A teenage male presents with obstructed nares and epistaxis. What should be suspected? And what is your treatement?**

Juvenile Nasopharyngeal Angiofibroma. Treated with embolizing the internal maxillary aa for control of bleeding then removal of the tumor.

○   *Inadvertent disruption of the auriculotemporal nerve during parotid surgery and subsequent cross-reinnervation with branches of the sympathetic supply to the skin may result in what syndrome?*

Frey's syndrome (postoperative gustatory sweating), seen after up to 50% of parotidectomies.

○   **What structures are preserved in the modified radical neck dissection?**

The sternocleidomastoid muscle, internal jugular vein and/or the spinal accessory nerve.

○   *Submandibular gland excision warrants careful dissection to prevent injury to what nerve?*

Marginal Mandibular Nerve.

○   **What is a ranula?**

A mucous retention cyst in the floor of the mouth characterized by a bluish surface.

○   *How should patients be followed after iodine 131 ablation post thyroidectomy for malignancy?*

Serum thyroglobulin levels.

○   *A 48 year old male presents with a high fever, trismus, dysphagia and swelling inferior to the mandible in the lateral neck. What is the most likely diagnosis?*

Parapharyngeal abscess.

○   **T/F: A patient can lose more of the upper lip than the lower lip without cosmetic problems.**

False. Up to one-third of the lower lip can be avulsed or debrided and the patient may still have an acceptable cosmetic appearance. The upper lip is less forgiving due to the relationship with the columella, alar bases and philtrum.

○   **Bilateral mental fractures may cause what acute complication?**

Airway obstruction.

❍   **What is the appropriate management of TMJ syndrome?**

Physiotherapy, analgesia, soft diet, muscle relaxants and warm moist compresses 4 to 5 times daily.

❍   **What structures are removed in the classic radical neck dissection?**

The sternocleidomastoid muscle, internal jugular vein, spinal accessory nerve and submandibular salivary gland with the associated lymph node-bearing fibrofatty tissue.

❍   **Where are most calculi within the parotid duct found?**

Near the orifice.

❍   *A pt is 1 month out from tracheostomy and has a small bleed from trach site. Then 24 hours later he has massive bleeding from the trach site. What is the problem?*

Tracheo/innominate fistula.

❍   **T/F: Tumors of the hypopharynx usual require laryngectomy.**

True.

❍   **How is the facial nerve best protected when performing operations on the parotid gland?**

By identifying its trunk as it exits the stylomastoid foramen at the posterior aspect of the gland.

❍   **What is the objective in performing a tympanoplasty?**

To improve sound pressure transmission to the oval window and to provide sound protection to the round window.

❍   *Patients with acoustic neuromas are more likely to complain of what symptom?*

Tinnitus and hearing loss.

❍   **T/F: Parapharyngeal abscesses should be drained through a transverse neck incision.**

True.

❍   **In which Le Fort fracture is CSF rhinorrhea most common?**

III.

❍   **A 16 year old boxer presents with right ear pain and swelling after receiving a blow to the ear. What is the appropriate treatment?**

The ear should be aseptically drained by incision or aspiration and a mastoid conforming dressing applied. ENT follow-up is mandatory.

❍   **A patient presents with a swollen, tender and erythematous left auricle. What is the most likely diagnosis?**

Perichondritis.

❍   **What physical findings are associated with a unilateral sensory hearing loss?**

The patient will have air conduction greater than bone conduction (normal Rinne test) and the Weber test will lateralize to the normal ear.

○   **What is the most common cause of unilateral sensory hearing loss?**

Viral neuronitis.

○   **What are the most common causes of bilateral sensory hearing loss?**

Noise or ototoxins such as certain antibiotics, loop diuretics and antineoplastics.

○   **A young male was involved in a bar room brawl and now complains of ear pain, significantly decreased hearing and vertigo. A tympanic membrane rupture is seen on exam. What is the major concern?**

Injury to the ossicles, temporal bone or labyrinth. Emergent ENT consult is necessary.

○   **What are the most common organisms causing acute otitis media in children?**

S. pneumoniae, Haemophilus influenza and Moraxella catarrhalis.

○   *In which salivary gland are stones most likely to occur?*

The submandibular gland.

○   **What percentage of patients with carcinoma of the tongue present with lymph node metastases?**

50%.

○   *What is the treatment of choice for a pleomorphic adenoma of the parotid gland?*

Superficial parotidectomy with preservation of the facial nerve.

○   **What is the most common cause of laryngeal trauma?**

Blunt trauma secondary to motor vehicle accidents.

○   **What x-ray findings are associated with lower airway foreign bodies?**

Air trapping on the affected side and a mediastinal shift to the contralateral side.

○   **What prophylaxis should be given to household contacts of patients with acute epiglottitis?**

Rifampin 20 mg/kg (maximum 600 mg) for 4 days.

○   **What is the treatment of choice for a radicular cyst of the mandible?**

Local excision or curettage.

○   **What means of airway maintenance are recommended for patients with Ludwig's angina?**

Tracheostomy or cricothyroidotomy.

○   **What is the most common indication for surgical drainage in patients with Ludwig's angina?**

Failure of antibiotic therapy.

❍ **What are the most common presenting signs of anterior lateral pharyngeal space infections?**

Trismus, swelling at the angle of the mandible and medial bulging of the pharyngeal wall.

❍ **What are the most common findings on lateral neck x-rays in patients with a retropharyngeal abscess?**

Prevertebral soft tissue widening, air-fluid levels, loss of cervical lordosis and cervical osteomyelitis.

❍ **What is the imaging modality of choice for the diagnosis of septic thrombophlebitis of the jugular vein?**

CT with contrast.

❍ **What are the most common bacterial causes of acute sinusitis?**

Pneumococcus and Haemophilus influenza.

❍ **What is the most common bacterial cause of malignant external otitis?**

Pseudomonas aeruginosa.

❍ **What is the most frequent neurological complication of malignant external otitis?**

Facial nerve palsy.

❍ **What antibiotic regimen is most appropriate in the treatment of malignant external otitis?**

Broad spectrum combination therapy with activity against Pseudomonas aeruginosa.

❍ **What is the most important risk factor for the development of acute bacterial parotitis?**

Dehydration.

❍ *What is the most common organism associated with acute suppurative parotitis?*

Staphylococcus aureus.

❍ **What is the treatment of choice for a patient with a peritonsillar abscess?**

Incision and drainage.

❍ **Through what anatomical space must a peritonsillar abscess extend to involve the carotid sheath?**

The lateral pharyngeal space.

❍ **What is the etiology of ventricular ectopy during right radical neck dissection?**

Trauma to the right stellate ganglion and cervical autonomic nervous system during dissection.

❍ **What is the mortality rate from hemorrhage following T & A?**

Between 1 in 4,000 and 1 in 27,000.

❍ **How long should a patient with epiglottitis remain intubated?**

36 to 48 hours (when inflammation has subsided).

○   **What is the treatment for croup?**

Humidified oxygen. If tachypnea and cyanosis are present, racemic epinephrine may be helpful.

○   **How is the diagnosis of sleep apnea syndrome confirmed?**

Complete cessation of airflow, oxygen desaturation to 90%, obstruction for 10 seconds or more with no air movement and paradoxical movement of the chest and abdomen or nasopharyngoscopic or cinofluoroscopic documentation of upper airway obstruction

○   *What sequelae result from superior laryngeal nerve injury?*

Loss of sensation above the vocal cords, impairment of laryngeal protective reflexes, hoarseness and limited vocalization of high-pitched tones (external branch).

○   *T/F: Atlantoaxial instability is more common in the pediatric population.*

True. The ligaments of the cervical spine are immature and loose and the odontoid process is not fully developed. (As many as 30% of children with Down's syndrome and achondroplastic dwarfism have atlantoaxial instability.)

○   **What complications are associated with surgery for head and neck cancer?**

Open neck veins can entrain air into the venous system, tumors involving the major vessels in the neck may require sacrifice of one or both internal jugular veins resulting in decreased cerebral perfusion pressure, cerebral edema and cardiac arrhythmias.

○   **What is the risk of general anesthesia in a patient with a peritonsillar abscess?**

Spontaneous rupture of the abscess with spillage of pus into an unprotected airway.

○   **T/F: In patients with cancer of the oral gingiva, extraction of a tooth in the area of the tumor provides access for rapid deep invasion of the bone.**

True.

○   **What are the indications for postoperative radiation therapy for the above patient?**

Massive tumor involvement, close or involved surgical margins, perivascular or perineural invasion and/or extensive nodal metastasis.

○   **T/F: The majority of minor salivary gland tumors in the upper aerodigestive tract are malignant.**

True, as opposed to the parotid gland in which the majority of tumors are benign.

○   **A patient presents with a small mass in the left parotid gland. FNA cytology shows SCC (squamous cell carcinoma). What is the likelihood that this is a primary SCC of the parotid?**

It is unlikely. Metastasis from the surrounding area is more common.

○   **T/F: Leukoplakia has a higher incidence of malignant transformation than erythroplakia.**

False.

○   **T/F: Non-epithelial cancers are the most prevalent malignancies in carcinoma of the larynx.**

False. Squamous cell carcinoma is the most common cancer (95 to 98%).

○ **On initial presentation of a patient with SCC arising in the tongue, floor of the mouth, gingiva or cheek mucosa, how many will have evidence of regional nodal metastasis?**

One-third.

○ **A patient presents with a complaint of a recurrent, painful swelling of the side of his face at mealtimes that usually resolves within 2 to 3 hours. What is the most likely diagnosis?**

Sialolithiasis.

○ **When does a mandible fracture become an airway embarrassment?**

If there are bilateral parasymphyseal fractures of the mandible.

○ **What signs and symptoms indicate malignancy of a parotid gland tumor?**

Weakness or paralysis of the facial nerve, presence of nodal enlargement and fixation of the tumor to skin or deep tissues.

○ **Which salivary gland tumor has a well-known propensity for extension along perineural spaces and invasion of bone?**

Adenoid cystic carcinoma.

○ **What are the common causes of stomal recurrence after laryngectomy?**

Submucosal extension of tumor, lymphatic spread, paratracheal lymph node metastasis and tumor implants at the site of surgery.

○ *A patient has undergone a total thyroidectomy for cancer. Postoperatively, the patient is unable to breathe after extubation. What surgical complication may have occurred?*

Bilateral recurrent laryngeal nerve injury.

○ *A toddler sustains an electrical injury to the commissure of his mouth after biting through an electrical cord from a floor lamp. What post-injury warning should be given to the parents?*

The labial artery may hemorrhage if the overlying soft tissue of the commissure breaks down. The parents should be instructed to hold digital pressure on the lip with their thumb and index finger to control the bleeding and seek help immediately.

○ **What is the most common intracranial complication of suppurative otitis media?**

Meningitis.

○ **An acutely ill child presents with profuse, purulent, foul smelling otorrhea and a large tympanic membrane perforation. What is the most likely diagnosis?**

Acute necrotizing otitis media caused by beta-hemolytic streptococcus.

○ **What are indications for myringotomy in acute otitis media?**

Failure of initial antibiotic therapy, severe pain, complicated acute otitis media and an immunocompromised patient.

O   **During a Valsalva maneuver, a weight lifter experiences sudden decrease in hearing with vertigo and unsteadiness. Over the next few weeks he has fluctuations in symptoms but with worsening hearing. What is the most likely diagnosis?**

A perilymphatic fistula.

O   **What distinguishes central from peripeheral facial nerve paralysis?**

Central has intact frontalis and orbicularis oculi function, intact mimetic function and absent Bell's phenomena.

O   **Which cranial nerve innervates derivatives of the second branchial arch?**

VII (geniculate ganglion).

O   **Fourth and sixth arch derivatives are innervated by which nerves?**

Superior laryngeal nerve and recurrent laryngeal nerve, respectively.

O   **In neonates, initial antibiotic therapy for acute otitis media should be effective against which organisms?**

Enteric organisms (gram negative).

O   **Nystagmus is defined by which component?**

Fast component. Slow phase is vestibular in origin, direction of endolymph flow; the fast phase is compensatory, from reticular formation.

O   **What is the most common result of delayed treatment of a septal hematoma?**

Cartilagenous necrosis with resultant saddle nose deformity.

O   **A 24 year old male presents with unilateral vigorous epistaxis following blunt trauma during a basketball game. His nasal dorsum is displaced laterally and intranasal examination reveals bleeding from the superior aspect of the nasal cavity. What is the most likely diagnosis?**

Traumatic injury to the anterior and posterior ethmoid arteries.

O   **What is the most important information to be gained from plain x-rays of the paranasal sinuses?**

Presence or absence of bony destruction.

O   *A 15 year old male presents to your office with persistent, severe and recurrent epistaxis associated with unilateral nasal obstruction. Examination reveals a large left-sided bluish intranasal mass. What is the most likely diagnosis?*

Juvenile angiofibroma.

O   **What signs and symptoms are associated with orbital blowout fractures?**

Diplopia with upward gaze, shallow supratarsal sulcus, enophthalmos and vertical shortening of the lower eyelid.

O   **What findings are associated with nasoethmoid fractures?**

The nose appears flattened with loss of dorsal nasal projection, nasolabial angle is obtuse, medial canthal areas are distorted, periorbital and subconjunctival hemorrhage are present, crepitance and loss of bone support are palpable and traumatic telecanthus. CSF rhinorrhea may also be present.

○ *What is the most common location of salivary gland tumors?*

The parotid gland (80%).

○ *What percentage of parotid gland tumors are malignant?*

20%.

○ *What is the most common malignant tumor of the parotid gland?*

Mucoepidermoid carcinoma.

○ *What is the most common malignant tumor of the submandibular gland?*

Adenoid cystic carcinoma.

○ *An 88 year old white male presents with a painless mass just below his ear that has been slowly enlarging over 2 to 3 years. Pathology shows round, plump, granular eosinophilic cells with small indented nuclei. What is the most likely diagnosis?*

Warthin's tumor (adenolymphoma), these tumors are bilateral 10% of the time.

○ **What is the most common bacterial pathogen causing cervical lymphadenitis in young children?**

Staphylococcus.

○ **The sensory distribution of which cranial nerves is responsible for the sensory distribution referred otalgia?**

CN V, IX and X.

○ **Which muscle is the sole abductor of the vocal cords?**

Posterior cricoarytenoid.

○ **A paralyzed vocal cord in the paramedian position is the result of what kind of injury?**

Isolated unilateral recurrent laryngeal nerve injury.

○ **Which intrinsic laryngeal muscles are responsible for tension of the vocal cords?**

Cricothyroid (chief tensor) and thyroarytenoid (internal tensor).

○ **What percentage of pediatric patients with laryngomalacia will also have subglottic stenosis?**

5%.

○ **What is the significance of vocal cord paralysis in a patient with thyroid cancer?**

Poor prognosis, neurapraxia due to compression, paralysis is not reversible and/or inoperability.

○ **A deep neck abscess secondary to pansinusitis will occur in which space?**

Retropharyngeal.

❍   **A 6 year old male presents with dysphagia, fever and noisy breathing. His voice is muffled when he speaks, his neck is stiff and he has rigid posturing of his head. What is the most likely diagnosis?**

Retropharyngeal abscess.

❍   **A 55 year old nonsmoking male presents with a sensation of a lump in his throat and constant throat clearing. He denies weight loss. The cough is most troublesome at night. Examination results are normal except for a moderately erythematous larynx, particularly in the posterior glottis. What would be the most effective initial management of this problem?**

Anti-reflux precautions.

❍   *Most branchial cleft cysts are found in which triangle of the neck?*

Anterior triangle, lateral to the midline

❍   *Where on the neck are most thyroglossal duct cysts found?*

Midline, beneath the hyoid and superior to the thyroid gland.

❍   **Where would you expect to find the parathyroid glands in a 10 year old patient with a lingual thyroid gland?**

In the tracheoesophageal groove.

❍   *A 3 year old boy presents with a midline anterior neck mass just below the hyoid bone that moves with deglutition and tongue protrusion. What is believed to be the cause of this congenital mass?*

Failure of complete obliteration of the thyroglossal duct.

❍   *An infant presents with coughing, choking and cyanosis during feeding. This clinical triad suggests what process?*

A tracheoesophageal fistula.

❍   **What are the most common sources of anterior epistaxis?**

Septal branches of the sphenopalatine artery and branches of the anterior ethmoidal and facial arteries.

❍   **What cranial nerves are most commonly affected by skull base lesions?**

CN VII and VIII.

❍   **What is the most common lesion of the cerebellopontine angle or skull base?**

Acoustic neuroma.

❍   **What is the most common initial finding in a patient with an acoustic neuroma?**

Unilateral sensorineural hearing loss.

❍   **What is the World Health Organization (WHO) classification of nasopharyngeal carcinomas (NPC)?**

Type 1 is keratinizing squamous cell carcinoma, type 2 is non-keratinizing squamous cell carcinoma and type 3 is undifferentiated carcinoma.

O **Which lip is most commonly affected by sun exposure-induced carcinoma?**

The lower lip.

O *What are the primary lymphatics for central lower lip cancer?*

The submental lymph nodes.

O *What is the most common histopathology for lip cancer?*

Squamous cell carcinoma.

O *What is the treatment of choice for lip cancer?*

Surgical excision.

O **What type of repair is required for defects at the oral commissure?**

An Estlander flap.

O **After lip cancer, what is the most common subsite for oral cancer?**

The oral tongue.

O **What is the most common cause of death in patients with advanced oral cancer?**

Locoregional failure.

O **What are the primary lymphatic zones at risk with oropharyngeal cancer?**

Zones II to IV (upper, middle and lower jugular lymph nodes).

O **What are the common symptoms of early oropharyngeal cancer?**

Dull ache in the throat, otalgia (ear pain) and globus sensation.

O **Which anatomic subdivision is most commonly involved in laryngeal cancer?**

The glottis.

O **What is the cure rate with radiation alone for T1 and T2 cancers of the larynx?**

80 to 95% for T1 cancers and 65 to 80% for T2 cancers.

O **Cancers of the supraglottis spread to which lymphatic groups?**

Zones II to IV (upper, middle and lower jugular nodes) bilaterally.

O **What syndrome is associated with post-cricoid carcinoma in non-smoking young women?**

Plummer-Vinson syndrome.

O **What anatomically divides Zones III and IV?**

The omohyoid muscle.

O   **What percentage of patients with parotid cancer will present with facial nerve paralysis?**

12%.

O   **What is the most significant prognostic variable in salivary gland cancer?**

Stage of the tumor at presentation.

O   *What is the incidence of gustatory sweating (Frey's syndrome) following parotidectomy?*

up to 50%.

O   **What is the incidence of cancer arising in a pre-existing benign pleomorphic adenoma?**

1.5% at 5 years, 10% at 15 years.

ESOPHAGUS, STOMACH, DUODENUM, AND GI PHYSIOLOGY PEARLS

Eat and drink measurely, and defy the mediciners.

Proverb

○ *What are the characteristic manometric findings in achalasia?*

Failure of the lower esophageal sphincter (LES) to relax completely with swallowing associated with an absence of organized propulsive peristalsis, elevated resting LES pressure and non-propulsive simultaneous contractions (tertiary waves).

○ **What is the most common complaint of patients with a duodenal ulcer?**

Epigastric pain.

○ **T/F: Elevated serum gastrin levels during fasting are typically seen in patients with a duodenal ulcer.**

False.

○ **What findings on esophagogastroduodenoscopy (EGD) and upper gastrointestinal (UGI) contrast studies are associated with achalasia?**

The bird beak esophagus is the classic UGI finding in achalasia. The gastroesophageal (GE) junction should not appear strictured and, except in end-stage cases, an adult endoscope should easily pass through the GE junction with steady pressure.

○ *What does the parietal cell secrete?*

HCL and Intrinsic Factor.

○ *What does intrinsic factor assist in?*

It binds to B12 and allows B12 absorbtion in the terminal ileum.

○ **What are the treatment options available to an otherwise healthy patient with achalasia?**

Endoscopic balloon dilation and operative (Heller) esophagomyotomy.

○ **An 80 year old man with severe achalasia, who is not a candidate for surgery, due to unrelated medical problems, requests treatment for his dysphagia. What is your recommendation?**

Botulinum injection.

○ **What major structures support the stomach?**

The gastrocolic, gastrosplenic and gastrophrenic ligaments.

O   **What is involved in the Belsey procedure?**

Two layers of plicating sutures placed between the gastric fundus and the lower esophagus with subsequent creation of a 280° anterior gastric wrap and posterior approximation of the crura.

O   *What is the best test to diagnose GERD?*

24 hour pH probe.

O   **What is the most important mechanism for maintenance of the GE junction?**

The intraabdominal segment of the esophagus.

O   *What is the treatment of choice for patients with primary achalasia?*

A modified Heller myotomy.

O   **Which cells produce pepsinogen?**

The chief cells produce pepsinogen which initiates gastric proteolysis.

O   **What peptide activates the digestive cascade?**

Enterokinase. Which then acts on trypsinogen to trypsin.

O   **A 70 year old man with a 30 year history of achalasia presents with recurrence of his symptoms after a successful balloon dilation several years previously. What is the appropriate treatment?**

Esophagomyotomy after carcinoma is ruled out.

O   **A 45 year old woman presents with manometrically documented primary achalasia. Her esophagus is massively dilated and contains a significant amount of undigested food. She has failed several prior attempts at modified Heller myotomies and has had several hospital admissions. What is the treatment of choice?**

Total esophagectomy.

O   **What are the potential intraoperative complications during transhiatal esophagectomy?**

Recurrent laryngeal nerve injury, tear in the membranous wall of the trachea, azygous vein disruption, hemothorax and pneumothorax.

O   **T/F: Stage for stage, the survival rate after radical en bloc esophagectomy is better than that after transhiatal esophagectomy.**

False.

O   **A patient with severe reflux symptoms has virtually complete relief with proton-pump inhibitor therapy. He still requests an operation so that he will not require medication. Is he a candidate for surgery?**

Yes. Surgery for gastroesophageal reflux (GER) is an option for patients who are concerned about the inconvenience, cost and long-term medical consequences of daily medication, provided the patient is medically fit for an operation.

❍ *How is GER most objectively documented?*

By 24-hour esophageal pH monitoring.

❍ **What is Barrett's esophagus?**

It refers to the presence of 2 to 3 cm of columnar epithelium along the esophageal mucosa. Alternatively, intestinal metaplasia is diagnostic of Barrett's, regardless of its proximal extent.

❍ **What is meant by a highly selective vagotomy?**

Division of individual branches of the nerve of Latarjet, preserving the crow's foot.

❍ **T/F: Esophageal manometry is a necessary part of the evaluation of a patient being considered for an anti-reflux condition.**

True.

❍ *What is the classic metabolic abnormality associated with gastric outlet obstruction?*

Hypochloremic, hypokalemic metabolic acidosis.

❍ *The best method of establishing the diagnosis of an esophageal leiomyoma is by what means, and what is the preferred treatment?*

Dx : typical appearance on EGD; TX : enucleation, NOT esophagectomy.

❍ **What is the most common type of gastric polyp?**

Hyperplastic polyps.

❍ **What is the criminal nerve of Grassi?**

A proximal branch of the posterior vagus nerve.

❍ **What are the three main peptides which act on the parietal cell ?**

Acetlycholine, Histamine and Gastrin which through calcium activate Protein kinase C, which then increases HCL secretion.

❍ **Which cells produce gastrin?**

G cells.. They are located in the antrum of the stomach. They are stimultated by amino acids and Acetylcystine. They are inhibited by acid.

❍ **Increase in gastrin levels are associated with what cell hyperplasia?**

Enterochromaffin hyperplasia.

❍ *What is secretin stimulation test?*

Test for gastrinoma. In normal pts the gasrin level goes down with administration of secretin. In gastrinoma, there is a paradoxical rise in serum gastrin levels with secretin administration.

❍ **Why do we do antrecomy for ulcer treatment?**

Removal of the G cells which are located in the antrum. And therefore remove Stimulation of G cells.

❍   *What happens to gastrin when pt takes Omeprizole?*

*First there is blocking of **H/K atpase** of parietal cell with a secondary decrease in acid production.*

❍   **A 50 year old otherwise healthy patient, who has suffered from recurrent lobar pneumonias, is referred for anti-reflux surgery. Under what circumstances would you be willing to operate?**

When GER can be objectively demonstrated on a 24-hour esophageal pH study. Evidence of reflux into the proximal esophagus, presence of laryngeal inflammation and a good response of pulmonary symptoms to a 3 month trial of high dose proton-pump inhibitors also correlates with a good response to surgery. Other etiologies for pulmonary symptoms must be eliminated.

❍   **A patient who underwent a Nissen fundoplication 2 weeks ago continues to have trouble swallowing. What is your recommendation?**

Allow time for the edema to resolve, then re-evaluate.

❍   **T/F: Traction diverticula are associated with tuberculosis.**

True.

❍   **What is a Schatzki's ring?**

A dense annular band in the submucosa at the squamocolumnar junction.

❍   **What is the most potent stimulant for gastric acid secretion?**

Ingestion of a mixed high-protein meal.

❍   **A patient whose reflux symptoms resolved following a Nissen fundoplication presents several years later with recurrent symptoms. What is the diagnostic test of choice?**

UGI contrast study.

❍   **A 45 year old patient with Barrett's esophagus, containing high grade dysplasia on endoscopic biopsy specimens from the distal esophagus, is referred to you. What is the treatment of choice?**

Total esophagectomy.

❍   **A 50 year old woman with a known reflux-induced stricture of the distal esophagus presents with dysphagia. She had successful endoscopic dilatation 1 year previously and was free of dysphagia until now. Her symptoms of GER are mild and controlled with H2 blockers as needed. How should she be managed?**

Malignancy must be ruled out prior to undertaking any therapy. Assuming her stricture is reflux-induced, repeat endoscopic dilation should successfully treat her dysphagia.

❍   **T/F: GER occurs in all patients with a sliding hiatal hernia.**

False.

❍   **What are the most common complications of type II hiatal hernias?**

Occult gastrointestintal bleeding, ulceration in the herniated portion of the stomach and gastric volvulus.

❍   **A patient with a long history of reflux symptoms presents with a peptic stricture of the distal esophagus that cannot be dilated by flexible or rigid endoscopy. What is the treatment of choice?**

Resection.

○   **What is the most important predictor of stomach ulcer recurrence?**

Slow healing of the initial ulcer (usually longer than 3 months).

○   **T/F: Routine splenectomy improves survival in patients with gastric adenocarcinoma.**

False.

○   **An 80 year old man presents with dysphagia that prevents him from adequately clearing his pharynx of food. He also notices gurgling in his neck when he swallows. What is the most likely diagnosis?**

A Zenker's diverticulum.

○   **What is the diagnostic test of choice for a Zenker's diverticulum?**

Barium swallow.

○   *What is the proper surgical approach for repair of a Zenker's diverticulum?*

A left lateral neck incision.

○   **Increased PTH is associated with what painful abdominal conditions?**

Gallstones and pancreatitis (it also will increase gastrin levels).

○   *What does Somatostatin do?*

It basically inhibits everything (it is a statin). It inhibits gastrin, insulin, secretin, Ach, and pancreatic and biliary output. It can be stimulated by acid in duodenum.

○   *What is the most common complicating symptom post vagotomy?*

Diarrhea.

○   *What are the types of dumping and the treatment?*

Early- due to hyperosmotic load. And fluid shifts.
Late- due to increase insulin and decrease glucose.
These both can usually be treated with dietary changes. 90% respond favorably to low carbohydrate loads.

○   *What is peptide YY role and where is it released?*

Released in terminal ileum and acts to inhibit acid secretion and GI motility.

○   *What is treatment of Gastric lymphoma?*

Chemoradiotherapy unless obstructing, perforated, or bleeding lesion.

○   *A 40 year old patient with a known history of alcohol abuse presents with a 6 hour history of severe epigastric pain following an episode of emesis. What is the appropriate initial diagnostic study in this patient's evaluation?*

UGI with water soluble contrast.

❍   The above patient's UGI study shows free flow of contrast from a perforation in the distal esophagus into the left pleural space. There are no other abnormalities. What is the treatment of choice?

Repair or replacement of his esophagus.

❍   *Under what circumstances is nonoperative management of an esophageal perforation appropriate?*

Minimal signs of systemic sepsis, the UGI shows no significant contamination of the pleural space and a sealed perforation, with all extravasated contrast returning to the lumen of the esophagus.

❍   A 40 year old woman suffers a laceration of her cervical esophagus during endoscopy. The laceration is recognized during the procedure and confirmed by a water-soluble contrast study. What is the appropriate treatment?

Drainage.

❍   An otherwise healthy patient with achalasia suffers an esophageal perforation during endoscopic balloon dilation of her LES. What is the appropriate management of this patient?

Repair the rent in conjunction with a modified Heller myotomy. A fundoplication may also be performed.

❍   A 65 year old patient is undergoing dilation for a peptic stricture of the distal esophagus when the esophagus is inadvertently perforated. How will you proceed?

The stricture must be resected, preferably through a transhiatal approach, with a cervical esophagogastrostomy.

❍   *A 50 year old otherwise healthy male presents with a spontaneous distal esophageal perforation into the left pleural space. He states that his epigastric pain began after an episode of vomiting 48 hours prior to his presentation. You perform a left lateral thoracotomy and the esophageal tissue around the site of perforation appears viable and will hold a suture. What is the treatment of choice?*

Primary repair of his esophagus.

❍   What is the most common malignant neoplasm of the esophagus?

Epidermoid cell cancer.

❍   T/F: Nissen Fundoplication can reverse the Barrett's metaplasia?

True, initially thought to only halt the progression of Barrett's, there is emerging evidence that fundoplication can actually reverse metaplasia.

❍   What is the best option for the above patient if on exploration, the esophageal tissue is too friable to confidently repair primarily?

Resection of the esophagus with a high thoracic or cervical esophagogastrostomy.

❍   A 34 year old female with documented GER and symptoms of severe heartburn, poorly controlled with proton-pump inhibitors, is referred for a Nissen fundoplication. On manometry, she has no peristalsis in the distal two-thirds of her esophagus and no identifiable LES. An UGI shows a moderately dilated esophagus with a patulous GE junction. She also complains of severe fatigue and very cold hands. What is the most likely diagnosis?

Scleroderma.

○ *What is the most appropriate treatment for a septic patient with a 48-hour-old perforation of the thoracic esophagus and pneumohydrothorax?*

Pleural drainage, esophageal exclusion, gastrostomy and cervical esophagostomy.

○ **What is the most common visceral complication secondary to cocaine use which requires abdominal exploration?**

Gastric ulcer. Bowel ischemia secondary to vasospasm is also well reported.

○ **What is the treatment of choice for the above patient?**

A Collis-Nissen procedure.

○ *What is the best modality to evaluate the T stage of esophageal and pancreatic tumors?*

Endoscopic ultrasound.

○ **What nonsurgical treatment options are most efficacious in the treatment of a patient with continuous bleeding from a Mallory-Weiss tear?**

Endoscopic cauterization or epinephrine injection of the bleeding site. When endoscopic modes of treatment fail, other options, such as balloon tamponade, angiographic embolization or intravenous pitressin infusion should be tried.

○ *What operation should be performed in a patient who continues to bleed from a Mallory-Weiss tear after endoscopic attempts to secure hemostasis have failed?*

The site of bleeding is oversewn, from within the lumen, through a high gastrotomy.

○ **What anatomic features of the esophagus render the transhiatal esophagectomy feasible?**

The thoracic esophagus is situated between organs in the mediastinum that have firm fascial or fibrous boundaries and is surrounded by loose areolar tissue, facilitating blunt dissection.

○ **What is the gastric output in patients with a duodenal ulcer?**

Approximately 40 mEq/l.

○ **Is postoperative NG tube after a low anterior resection of the rectum for adenocarcinoma is beneficial ?**

No.

○ *How does erythromycin stimulate the GI tract?*

It acts on the motilin receptor and is prokinetic. Motilin is the key stimulatory Hormone of the MMC.

○ *What does the most water absorption occur?*

Jejunum.

○ **A 70 year old patient has an early esophageal adenocarcinoma 39 cm from the incisors, involving only the submucosa. There is no apparent nodal involvement on endoscopic ultrasound. He has an FEV1 of 0.7 but is otherwise in good health. Assuming the remainder of his staging studies do not reveal disseminated disease, what is his best surgical option?**

A transhiatal esophagectomy.

O   **A patient has an esophageal tumor invading the muscularis propria and all lymph nodes are free of tumor. What stage is this patient's disease?**

Stage IIA.

O   **How can severe bile reflux esophagitis, refractory to medical treatment, be surgically managed?**

Gastric fundoplication.

O   **A 70 year old man presents with an upper thoracic esophageal cancer that impinges on the trachea. There is no sign of disseminated disease on the CT scan or other staging studies. What is the optimal surgical approach for this patient?**

Combined right thoracotomy and upper midline laparotomy.

O   **T/F: Intrathoracic anastomotic esophago-gastrostomy leak post esophagectomy does not always mandate surgical exploration?**

True, if external drainage is maintained without signs of sepsis or local tissue necrosis, conservative treatment with a distal feeding tube (J) can be used.

O   **How does the GB concentrate bile?**

Active reabsorption of NA, CL with water absorption via osmosis. The bile pool is 5g and it is recirculated every 4 hrs and we lose .5gm daily.

O   **A 65 year old man presents with squamous cell carcinoma of the esophagus extending from 34 to 40 cm from the incisors. On endoscopic ultrasound there are several hypoechoic, non-homogenous, sharply delineated paraesophageal lymph nodes within the mediastinum that are 2 cm in diameter. There are no signs of disseminated disease on this or additional staging studies. What is the best surgical approach for this lesion?**

A left thoracoabdominal incision.

O   **Which organ is most commonly used for reconstruction in the above scenario?**

The stomach.

O   **What is the procedure of choice for Type II or III gastric ulcers?**

Billroth I or II.

O   **What are the primary and secondary bile acids?**

Primary- Cholic and chenodeoxycholic acid.
Secondary-Deoxycholic acid and Lithocholic acid.

O   *What are the occurances of dumping and ulcer recurrence in Selective vagotomy, Truncal Vagotomy and Truncal Vagotomy and Antrectomy?*

	Dumping	Recurrence
SV	1%	15%
TV	10%	10%
TV+A	15%	1%

❍   **You plan to perform a near-total esophagectomy through a left thoracoabdominal incision with a cervical esophagogastrostomy for a low lying esophageal cancer. Will the patient require ablation of his pylorus?**

Not routinely. However, he may later require a pyloroplasty or pyloromyotomy.

❍   **A patient who had previously undergone a vagotomy and antrectomy for peptic ulcer disease (PUD) presents with a midthoracic esophageal squamous cell carcinoma. Assuming he is a candidate for curative resection, what is the best choice for reconstruction?**

The colon.

❍   **A patient with an adenocarcinoma of the gastroesophageal (GE) junction is seen on CT scan and endoscopic ultrasound to have several suspicious lymph nodes surrounding the left gastric artery. Is this patient a candidate for curative resection?**

Yes.

❍   **During the course of a planned curative esophagectomy for an obstructing adenocarcinoma of the esophagus 38 cm from the incisors, malignant adenopathy is discovered in the hepatoduodenal ligament. The tumor does not involve any mediastinal structures on preoperative staging studies. Should esophagectomy still be considered.**

Yes.

❍   *What is the strongest cell layer in the esophagus?*

The mucosa. (Remember there is not serosa layer in esophagus.)

❍   *What type of hiatal hernia is always managed surgically?*

Paraesophageal.

❍   *What is the treatment of Zenker's diverticulum?*

Myotomy and diverticulectomy.

❍   **What are the most common locations for an ectopic pancreas?**

The gastric antrum or duodenum.

❍   **What is the most common malignant tumor of the duodenum?**

Adenocarcinoma.

❍   *What is the initial procedure for a patient with Zollinger-Ellison syndrome and hyperparathyroidism?*

Parathyroidectomy.

❍   *What are the normal components of Bile?*

Bile salts-80%.
Lecithin-15%.
Cholesterol-5% - patients with increased cholesterol concentration form stones.

❍   **What is the treatment for patients with locally extensive cancers of the cervical esophagus?**

Surgery is usually required for effective palliation. It requires resection of the cervical esophagus and the larynx. Reconstruction involves a cervical tracheal stoma and completion blunt esophagectomy with a pharyngoesophagostomy.

O   **A 65 year old male with a known upper thoracic esophageal squamous cell carcinoma presents with paroxysmal coughing with meals. What is the most likely diagnosis?**

Malignant tracheoesophageal fistula.

O   **What is the best palliative treatment for the above patient?**

Esophageal stenting.

O   **What are the most important mediators of hydrochloric acid release?**

Histamine, acetylcholine and gastrin.

O   *A 56 year old male underwent resection of a midthoracic esophageal tumor through a combined right thoracotomy and midline laparotomy and a high intrathoracic anastomosis was performed. He subsequently developed high fevers and right-sided chest pain. A gastrograffin swallow shows a small leak at the anastomosis. What is the appropriate treatment?*

The right chest must be re-explored. If the conduit is viable, the leak may be buttressed with mediastinal tissue or an intercostal muscle flap and drained. If the conduit is ischemic or gangrenous, it must be resected, the intrathoracic esophagus oversewn and a diverting cervical esophagostomy performed.

O   **A patient with a locally extensive midthoracic esophageal squamous cell carcinoma has multiple pulmonary metastases on a CT scan of the chest. He has severe dysphagia and would like to be able to eat and drink again. What is the treatment of choice?**

Endoscopic stent placement or laser therapy.

O   **T/F: Adjuvant chemotherapy and radiation have no role in the treatment of esophageal tumors that are potentially resectable for cure.**

False.

O   **What are the manometric criteria for diffuse esophageal spasm (DES)?**

Frequent simultaneous contractions associated with normal LES function and normal peristaltic contractions.

O   *A pt has problem swallowing. A barium swallow is ordered showing a birds beak and manomerty is done showing lack of peristalsis and elevated LES pressures. What is your diagnosis? What is your treatment?*

Achalasia. Treatment is laparoscopic or open heller myotomy.

O   *T/F: Barretts esophagus is metaplasia from columnar to squamous cells?*

False. Metaplasia from squamous to columnar.

O   **What is the most common type of esophageal cancer in the united states?**

Adeno CA.

O   **During esophagectomy which vessel do you not want to cut. It will serve as a the blood supply to the pulled up stomach?**

Right Gastroepiploic.

O   **Under what circumstances is surgery warranted for DES?**

Severe symptoms and failed nitrate or calcium channel blocker therapy.

O   **What is the surgical treatment of DES?**

An extended esophageal myotomy.

O   **A 2 year old male has a dime lodged in his esophagus at the level of the cricopharyngeus. What is the treatment of choice?**

Endoscopic extraction.

O   *After undergoing a seeming uncomplicated laparoscopic Nissen fundoplication, a 42 year old man develops shortness of breath in the recovery room. What surgical complication is most likely?*

Iatrogenic pneumothorax.

O   **What is the most appropriate treatment for symptomatic duodenal diverticula?**

Surgical excision.

O   **How should button batteries lodged in the esophagus be treated?**

Emergency endoscopic removal. An upper gastrointestinal contrast study should be obtained the following day and within several weeks to assess for perforation and stricture formation.

O   **A 65 year old male has a large opacity in the anteromedial aspect of the right thorax on a routine chest x-ray. The opacity appears to have air within it. The patient is asymptomatic and has not had a previous chest x-ray. What is the most likely diagnosis?**

A foramen of Morgagni hernia.

O   *During the course of a radiologic contrast examination of the UGI tract, performed for abdominal pain, a 3 cm nonobstructing lesion, that appears to be a leiyomyoma, is discovered. The patient denies chest pain, dysphagia or heartburn. What is your recommendation?*

Enucleation.

O   **A 70 year old female with dysphagia has a large epiphrenic diverticulum on an UGI contrast study. What is the treatment of choice?**

Resection of the diverticulum with contralateral myotomy and fundoplication.

O   *What is the best initial treatment for a paraesphageal hiatal hernia?*

Surgical repair, transabdominally.

O   **What is the initial workup for a patient who presents following recent ingestion of a caustic substance?**

History and early endoscopy.

O   **What are the indications for surgery in the acute setting of caustic ingestion?**

Free air under the diaphragm, cervical crepitus and full-thickness necrosis of the esophagus or stomach.

○   **T/F: The majority of patients with hiatal hernias have clinically significant GER.**

False.

○   *What is the treatment of choice for traumatic disruption of the diaphragm?*

Repair via abdominal approach.

○   **What is the position of the GE junction when a paraesophageal hernia is present?**

Below the diaphragm (normal position).

○   *What is the treatment for Crohn's disease with numerous strictures?*
Multiple stricturoplasties when possible, the goal of surgery in regional enteritis is to conserve as much bowl as possible due to the relapsing/remitting nature of the disease along the entire GI tract.

○   **What metabolite is found in the urine of pts with carcinoid syndrome?**

5HIAA.

○   **What factors make gastrointestinal fistulas less likely to heal? (FRIENDS)**

Foreign body
Radiation
IBD or **I**nfection
Epithelization
Neoplasm
Distal obstruction
Sepsis

○   **What are the most common complications of paraesophageal hernias?**

Chronic blood loss anemia and gastric volvulus.

○   **What disorders of the esophagus are associated with the development of esophageal carcinoma?**

Lye ingestion, achalasia, Barrett's esophagus and Plummer-Vinson syndrome.

○   **What are the most important determinants of survival after resection of an esophageal carcinoma?**

Depth of invasion, the presence or absence of lymph node metastases and the presence or absence of distant metastases.

○   **Transmural involvement of an esophageal carcinoma suggests what T stage?**

T3.

○   **In addition to a CT scan of the chest and abdomen, what is included in the preoperative evaluation of proximal and upper mid-esophageal cancer?**

Bronchoscopy.

○   **What is the best surgical approach for resection of a bulky esophageal carcinoma 25 cm from the incisors?**

The Ivor-Lewis approach.

○   **What is the most appropriate treatment for a patient with epidermolysis bullosa, mild chest pain, low grade fever and minimal mediastinal involvement?**

Antibiotics, NPO and parenteral nutrition.

○   **What is the 5-year survival rate of a patient following complete resection of a stage II adenocarcinoma of the esophagus?**

25%.

○   **T/F: Adjuvant chemotherapy and/or radiotherapy improves the survival of a completely resected N1 esophageal carcinoma.**

False.

○   **What are the complications of a prolonged chylous leak?**

Lymphopenia, immunosuppression, malnutrition, loss of proteins, fats and fat soluble vitamins, dehydration and electrolyte loss.

○   **What is the main risk of radiation therapy in patients with an unresectable mid-esophageal cancer that involves the left main stem bronchus?**

The creation of a bronchoesophageal fistula.

○   **T/F: Induction radiation therapy followed by surgery improves the survival of esophageal cancer over that obtained by surgery alone.**

False.

○   **T/F: Combination chemoradiotherapy is superior to radiation therapy alone in the treatment of non-metastatic esophageal cancer.**

True.

○   **T/F: Combination induction chemotherapy and radiation, followed by surgery, improves 5-year survival compared to surgery alone, in resectable esophageal cancer.**

True.

○   *What is the most significant prognostic variable for a small bowel leiomyosarcoma devoid of any evidence of metastasis?*

Tumor grade.

○   **What is the difference between the muscle layers of the proximal and distal stomach?**

The smooth muscle of the proximal stomach is electrically stable, whereas the smooth muscle of the distal stomach shows spontaneous repeating electrical discharges. Pacesetter potentials originate along the greater curvature at a point in the proximal third of the stomach and fire at a rate of 3/min, initiating a peristaltic wave. There are no pacesetters or action potentials in the proximal stomach.

○   **What is the most common location of a stomach ulcer?**

The lesser curvature, near the incisura angularis (type 1).

O   **What are medical options to assist in closing a non-healing enero-enteic fistula secondary to Crohn's disease?**

Anti-TNF antibody or antimetabolites (methotrexate and azathioprine).

O   **Which type of stomach ulcer is associated with the highest level of hydrochloric acid production?**

Patients with combined gastric and duodenal ulcers (Type II) and with pre-pyloric ulcers (Type III).

O   **What is the incidence of colonization with Helicobacter pylori in the adult population?**

At least 50%.

O   **What are the indications for elective surgical treatment of a benign gastric ulcer?**

Failure to heal within 12 weeks of medical therapy, recurrence after 2 initial courses of successful treatment or inability to exclude malignancy.

O   **What are the surgical options for patients with a gastric ulcer?**

Vagotomy and drainage, vagotomy and antrectomy, vagotomy and subtotal gastrectomy, total gastrectomy and gastric devascularization.

O   **What are the most prominent postgastrectomy syndromes?**

Dumping syndrome and alkaline reflux gastritis are the most frequent. Other syndromes include diarrhea, afferent loop, blind loop, malabsorption, recurrent ulcer and bezoar.

O   **What is the drug of choice for the treatment of duodenal ulcers in pregnant women?**

Sucralfate.

O   **What is the most common side effect of misoprostol?**

Diarrhea.

O   **What is the effect of vagotomy on gastric acid output?**

It reduces acid secretion by about 80% in the immediate postoperative period and diminishes parietal cell responsiveness to gastrin and histamine.

O   **What are the criteria for definitive versus delayed repair of a perforated ulcer?**

If there has been no preoperative shock or life-threatening coexisting medical illness and the perforation has been present for less than 48 hours, a definitive ulcer operation may be performed. If these criteria are not met, immediate simple omental patching is usually safer.

O   **What is the lifetime risk of obstruction from an untreated peptic ulcer?**

10%.

O   **What is the treatment of choice for patients with alkaline reflux gastritis?**

Roux-en-Y gastrojejunostomy with an intestinal limb of 50 to 60 cm.

O   **What are the most frequent long-term postoperative complications of jejuno-ileal bypass?**

Cirrhosis, cholelithiasis, nephrolithiasis, severe fluid and electrolyte abnormalities and development of specific vitamin and micronutrient deficiencies.

❍   **What is the most feared complication of gastric surgery for morbid obesity?**

Postoperative gastric leak and subsequent development of peritonitis.

❍   **What is the most common organism found in the mucosa of patients with stomach disorders?**

Helicobacter pylori.

❍   **What is the most common symptom of progression of gastric cancer?**

Pain.

❍   **What is the histologic appearance of the intestinal form of gastric carcinoma?**

A gland-like structure of the malignant cells.

❍   **What is the most common site of gastrointestinal lymphomas?**

The stomach.

❍   **What is the most common sarcoma of the stomach?**

Leiomyosarcoma.

❍   **What is the treatment of choice for gastric sarcomas?**

Gastrectomy.

❍   **A patient with known reflux esophagitis, on H2-antagonist therapy, presents for routine endoscopic follow-up. EGD reveals linear ulcerations of the distal esophagus without evidence of coalescence. What grade of esophagitis is present?**

Grade II.

❍   **What is the most common site of esophageal perforation in Boerhaave's syndrome?**

The left posterolateral esophagus, 3 to 5 cm above the GE junction.

❍   **What is the etiology of stress gastritis?**

A defective gastric mucosal barrier.

❍   **What is the most common factor predisposing patients in the critical care setting to stress gastritis?**

Decreased gastric mucosal blood flow due to inadequate perfusion.

❍   **What is the incidence of malignancy in gastric ulcers?**

15 to 25%.

❍   **What is the incidence of H. pylori infection in gastric ulcers?**

75%.

❍   **T/F: Type I gastric ulcers are frequently complicated by hemorrhage.**

False.

❍   **How often is metastatic disease present on initial diagnosis of gastric carcinoma?**

15%.

❍   *How extensive should surgical margins be to decrease risk of recurrence in resection for gastric carcinoma?*

5 or 6 cm.

❍   **Histologically, what is the similarity between Chaga's disease and achalasia?**

A decrease in the number of ganglion cells in Auerbach's plexus.

❍   **What gastric neuroendocrine tumor is more commonly seen in patients with pernicious anemia?**

Carcinoid.

❍   **T/F: In resecting a gastric leiomyosarcoma, lymphadenectomy is routinely indicated.**

False.

APPENDIX AND INGUINAL HERNIAS PEARLS

The patient suffered from chronic remunerative appendicitis.
Dilbert H. Nickson

○ **What percentage of gangrenous appendices are associated with a fecalith?**

Two-thirds.

○ **What is the most frequent site of rupture of the appendix?**

The antimesenteric border.

○ **In a pregnant woman in her third trimester, where is the pain of appendicitis most likely to occur?**

In the epigastric region or in the right upper quadrant.

○ **Where can a pelvic abscess resulting from appendicitis be drained?**

Through the rectum or vagina.

○ **When should appendectomy be performed when an appendiceal abscess is identified and drained?**

6 to 8 weeks after drainage, if appendectomy not performed initially.

○ **What is the most common cause of appendiceal stump or cecal rupture after appendectomy?**

Enema administration.

○ **How often is the appendix affected in endometriosis?**

1%.

○ **What percentage of all appendices harbor carcinoid tumor?**

0.1%.

○ **What is the distribution of carcinoid in the appendix?**

71% at the tip, 22% in the body and 7% at the base.

○ *What is the treatment for a carcinoid tumor that is less than 2 cm in size, is located at the tip of the appendix and has no evidence of nodal spread?*

Appendectomy.

○ *What is the treatment for a carcinoid tumor that is less than 2 cm in size, is located at the tip of the appendix and has evidence of nodal spread?*

Right hemicolectomy.

O   *What is the treatment for a carcinoid tumor of the appendix that is greater than 2 cm?*

Right hemicolectomy.

O   **When does appendiceal lymphoid tissue reach its peak level?**

In the teens.

O   **What is the negative appendectomy rate in appendicitis?**

10 to 20%.

O   *What is the treatment of adenocarcinoma of the appendix?*

Right hemicolectomy.

O   **What is the origin of the sympathetic nervous supply to the appendix?**

The superior mesenteric plexus.

O   **What is the most common cause of appendiceal lumen obstruction in children and young adults?**

Lymphoid hyperplasia from submucosal follicles.

O   **What is the most common cause of recurrence following indirect hernia repair?**

Inadequate repair of the inguinal floor.

O   **What percentage of appendicitis is associated with lymphoid hyperplasia?**

60%.

O   **What area of the appendix has the poorest blood supply?**

The midportion of the antimesenteric border.

O   **What systemic diseases can cause lymphoid hyperplasia in the appendix?**

Gastroenteritis from shigella and salmonella, upper respiratory tract infections, infectious mononucleosis and measles.

O   **What are the borders of the femoral canal?**

The iliopubic tract superiorly and medially, Cooper's ligament inferiorly and the femoral vein laterally.

O   **What percentage of appendicitis in adults is caused by a fecalith?**

30%.

O   *During surgery for presumed appendicitis, the appendix is found to be normal. However, the terminal ileum has an appearance consistent with Crohn's disease. Should appendectomy still be performed?*

Yes.

O   **What is the mortality rate for nonperforated appendicitis?**

Up to 0.6%.

○   **What is the mortality rate for perforated appendicitis?**

Up to 5%.

○   **What is the hypothesized sequence of events in appendicitis?**

Luminal obstruction → mucous accumulation → increased intraluminal pressure → local bacteria convert the mucous to pus → further increase in intraluminal pressure → lymphatic obstruction → edema of the appendix → diapedesis of bacteria → mucosal ulcers → venous obstruction → ischemia of the appendix → bacteria spread through the abdominal wall → acute suppurative appendicitis.

○   **What percentage of patients with acute appendicitis have atypical abdominal pain?**

Approximately 45%.

○   **What is the typical core temperature seen in patients with acute appendicitis?**

Normal to 38° C.

○   **What percentage of patients with acute appendicitis have a normal WBC count?**

30%.

○   **What is the reverse 3 sign?**

An extrinsic filling defect in the cecum.

○   **What ultrasound findings are consistent with acute appendicitis?**

Diameter greater than 6 mm, noncompressibility of the appendix and presence of a complex mass.

○   **What is the rate of perforation in appendicitis in children less than 1 year old? Less than 5 years old?**

100% and 50%, respectively.

○   **What is the overall negative laparotomy rate for suspected appendicitis?**

Traditionally 20%, although this is decreasing with more frequent use of CT scanning.

○   **What is the incidence of appendicitis in pregnancy?**

1 in 2000 pregnancies.

○   **What percentage of patients with unperforated appendicitis have complications?**

5%.

○   **What are the most common organisms found in wound infections after appendectomy?**

Bacteroides, klebsiella, enterobacter and E. coli.

○   **What is the most common cause of intestinal obstruction world wide?**

Hernias.

○   **What is the sex distribution of inguinal hernias?**
Male:female is 7:1.

○   **What is the incidence of the different hernias?**

Inguinal hernias (80%), umbilical hernias (14%) and femoral hernias (5%) . The remaining are rare.

○   **What is the probability of having an inguinal hernia in a patient with a femoral hernia?**

50% in men and 10% in women.

○   **What is the difference between the linea semicircularis and the linea semilunaris?**

The linea semicircularis is the lower edge of the posterior rectus sheath, about 3 to 6 cm below the level of umbilicus. The linea semilunaris (line of Douglas) is the curved depression seen lateral to the rectus abdominis muscle.

○   **What is the obturator sign?**

Pain on internal rotation of the right hip.

○   *Where does a Spigelian hernia occur?*

Through the linea semilunaris, lateral to the rectus muscles and inferior to the linea semicircularis, beneath the external oblique muscle.

○   **What is a Richter's hernia and why is it dangerous?**

One in which the contents includes one side (usually the antimesenteric side) of the intestinal wall. This hernia strangulates without any evidence of intestinal obstruction and is, therefore, easy to miss.

○   **What is the mortality rate of ruptured appendices in the elderly?**

15%.

○   **What is a sliding hernia?**

One in which part of the wall of the sac consists of a viscus (e.g., urinary bladder, cecum, etc.).

○   **What is the triangle of doom?**

The area between the vas deferens and the gonadal vessels seen on the laparoscopic approach where, for example, the iliac vessels are at risk of injury from staples.

○   **What is Amyand's hernia?**

The hernia sac contains a ruptured appendix. This is usually mistaken for a strangulated hernia.

○   **What is the appropriate management for a ruptured appendix?**

Drainage with prompt appendectomy or interval appendectomy if the appendix cannot be safely removed. In addition, perioperative antibiotics against aerobic and anaerobic bacteria should be continued until no evidence of infection or abscess is present.

○   **T/F: The incidence of acute appendicitis is increased in pregnant women.**

False.

○ **T/F: Acute appendicitis is the most common cause of an acute abdomen in pregnant women past the first trimester.**
True.

○ **What structures are derived from the external oblique muscle and its aponeurosis?**

The inguinal ligament, lacunar ligament and the superficial inguinal ring.

○ **What is the most common vascular structure injured during groin hernia repair?**

The femoral artery.

○ **What is Littre's hernia?**

An inguinal hernia with an incarcerated Meckel's diverticulum.

○ **What are the boundaries of the internal inguinal ring?**

Arching fibers of the transversus abdominis and internal oblique muscles superomedially and the iliopubic tract inferolaterally.

○ **Why is the right side twice as prone to develop an inguinal or a femoral hernia compared to the left?**

The right testis descends into the scrotum later than the left. The processus vaginalis is, therefore, patent for a longer period and atrophies later than the left side. In addition, the sigmoid colon on the left side protects against possible herniation.

○ **What is the appropriate treatment for an incidental carcinoid tumor with tumor found at the surgical margins?**

Right hemicolectomy.

○ **What are the boundaries of the superior lumbar triangle of Grynfelt?**

The superior border is the 12th rib, the inferior border is the internal oblique muscle and the posterior border is the sacrospinalis muscle.

○ **What are the boundaries of the inferior lumbar triangle of Petit?**

The posterior border is the lattisimus dorsi, the anterior border is the external oblique and the inferior border is the iliac crest.

○ **What is the origin of the genital branch of the genitofemoral nerve and what does it supply?**

It arises from L1 and L2, supplies motor fibers to the cremasteric muscle and is the sensory supply to the side of the scrotum and labia.

○ **What is the mortality rate when a hernia becomes strangulated?**

10%.

○ **When is expectant treatment for a hernia appropriate?**

When the morbidity or mortality of the procedure, due to concomitant disease, exceeds that of potential complications. Most of the small umbilical hernias in children close spontaneously by 2 years of age and can, therefore, be observed. An asymptomatic ventral hernia with no sign of incarceration may also be observed.

○   **What does the McVay repair entail?**

Approximation of the transverse abdominus aponeurosis to Cooper's ligament.

○   **What is the appropriate treatment of an appendiceal mucocele found during abdominal surgery?**

Appendectomy.

○   **Where is local anesthesia administered for inguinal hernia repair?**

For the ilioinguinal nerve block, the anesthesia is given 2 cm medial to the anterior superior iliac spine and the skin is then infiltrated along the line of incision. After opening the inguinal canal, further local anesthesia can be given at the following sites: around the internal ring, in the loose areolar tissue around the spermatic cord, near the internal ring, at the neck of the sac and over the pubic tubercle.

○   **What type of hernia is most likely to recur?**

An incisional hernia.

○   **What is a Lichtenstein repair?**

A tension-free replacement of the transveralis fascia with nonabsorbable mesh.

○   **What are the advantages of laparoscopic hernia repair?**

It is useful for bilateral or recurrent hernias, causes less pain, early return to work and better cosmesis.

○   **What is a Tanner' slide?**

The relaxing incision in the transversus abdominis, superomedial to the inguinal canal, to relieve tension on the repair.

○   **What are the local complications of an inguinal hernia repair?**

Wound infections, hematomas, sinus and fistula formation, orchitis, testicular atrophy, injury to the vas deferens, hydrocele, sensory and motor nerve damage, postoperative pain, vascular injuries to the femoral or testicular vessels, bladder or bowel injuries and recurrence.

○   **What is the reported recurrence rate after an inguinal hernia repair?**

Classsically, it is thought to be 5 to 10% for indirect inguinal hernias, 10 to 15% for direct inguinal hernias and 30% for recurrent inguinal hernias; however, the addition of synthetic meshes have dramatically reduced these recurrence rates.

○   **What is the recurrence rate after an incisional hernia repair?**

30%, this also has been reduced to less than 10% with the advent of mesh.

○   **What are the technical reasons for the high recurrence rate after incisional hernia repair?**

Wound infection, inadequate dissection with poor exposure, closure under tension and failure to include other hernial orifices adjacent to the main hernia.

○   **What is the incidence of epigastric hernias?**

5%. Male:female is 2:1.

○ **What is the usual content of epigastric hernias?**

Preperitoneal fat.

○ **What is the relationship of a single midline decussation of rectus to abdominal hernias?**

80% of the umbilical hernias and almost all epigastric hernias occur in patients who have a single decussation (30% of the population).

○ **T/F: The incidence of umbilical hernias is different in African Americans and Caucasians.**

True. 40 to 90% of African American infants are born with an umbilical hernia compared to 20% of Caucasian infants.

○ **What are the signs of impending rupture of an umbilical hernia?**

Discoloration, ulceration or rapid increase in size.

○ **What is the relationship between interparietal hernias and maldescent of the testis?**

Interparietal hernias are almost exclusively right sided and 70% are associated with a maldescended or ectopic testis.

○ **During an obturator hernia repair, where can the obturator membrane be incised to avoid injury to the obturator vessels?**

At the inferior margin.

○ **What is the sex ratio of obturator hernias?**

Male:female is 1:5.

○ **What is the Howship Romberg sign?**

Pain passing down the inner side of the thigh to the knee in an obturator hernia.

○ **What are the 3 types of sciatic hernias?**

Through the greater sciatic notch there are 2 variants: suprapiriformis (60%) and infrapiriformis (30%) and through the lesser sciatic foramen is the subspinous (10%).

○ **What is Laugier's (Velpeau's) hernia?**

A hernia through the lacunar ligament.

○ **What is a Cooper's hernia?**

The hernia sac follows the femoral canal but tracks down to the scrotum, labia majorus or the obturator foramen.

○ **What is a prevascular hernia?**

When the hernia is in front of the external iliac vessels within the femoral sheath.

CARDIAC SURGERY PEARLS

No man really becomes a fool until he stops asking questions.
Charles Steinmetz

○ **What is the most common cause of pulmonary hypertension in children?**

Persistence of fetal histology in the pulmonary arteries.

○ **What percentage of adults have a patent foramen ovale?**

10 to 20%.

○ **When do intracardiac shunts become physiologically important?**

When the pulmonary blood flow exceeds 1.5 to 2 times the systemic flow.

○ **Why is a paradoxical embolus able to cause septic end-organ disease?**

An infected venous thrombus can enter the arterial circulation via a right-to-left intracardiac shunt and be sent distal to affect end-organs.

○ **T/F: Increased pulmonary blood flow and congestion increase the susceptibility to bacterial infection.**

True.

○ **T/F: Tissue valves are longer lasting than mechanical valves.**

False. They are shorter acting, but have the benefit of not needing anticoagulation therefore they are ideal in pts with contraindications to anticoagulation.

○ **What type of intracardiac shunt is most frequently associated with pulmonary hypertension?**

A ventricular septal defect (VSD).

○ **What radiographic finding is associated with transposition of the great vessels?**

An egg-shaped heart.

○ **What are the pathophysiologic consequences of a left-to-right intracardiac shunt?**

Diastolic overloading, cardiac dilatation and ventricular enlargement.

○ **What is the most important parameter in the evaluation of patients with pulmonary hypertension?**

The pulmonary vascular resistance.

○ **T/F: Congestive heart failure (CHF) usually develops in children with a right-to-left intracardiac shunt.**

False.

○   *What are the two types of aortic dissection and their management?*

Type A- Proximal to L subclavian- Surgical.
Type B- Distal to L sublavian- Medical with aggressive HTN control.

○   **What factors affect the degree of cyanosis in patients with a right-to-left intracardiac shunt?**

The severity of anoxia and the concentration of blood hemoglobin.

○   **Left atrial enlargement is associated with which congenital heart defects?**

Mitral insufficiency, patent ductus arteriosus (PDA) and VSD.

○   **What auscultatory finding is associated with PDA?**

A widely split and fixed S2.

○   **Which congenital heart defects are associated with congenital aortic stenosis?**

PDA, VSD, coarctation of the aorta and mitral valve defects.

○   **T/F: ECG accurately determines the severity of obstruction in patients with pulmonic stenosis.**

True.

○   **Splinter hemorrhages, Osler's nodes, Janeway lesions, petechiae and Roth's spots can be indications of what process?**

Infective endocarditis.

○   **What percentage of patients with infective endocarditis display peripheral manifestations of the disease?**

50%.

○   **How is bacterial endocarditis diagnosed?**

Evidence of valvular vegetations on echocardiogram combined with a positive blood culture.

○   **If patients have not yet received antibiotics, what percentage of culture negative endocarditis is expected?**

Less than 5%.

○   *When does the Intra Aortic Balloon Pump inflate?*

Inflates during diastol before the T wave and deflates with p wave.

○   *How does IABP assist cardiac output?*

It increases coronary blood flow and reduces afterload by inflating during diastole.

○   **What is the sensitivity of a two-dimensional transesophageal echocardiogram for detecting vegetations?**

95%.

○ **Who is at high risk for developing endocarditis?**

Patients with prosthetic heart valves, previous incidents of endocarditis, complex congenital heart disease, intravenous drug use and surgically devised systemic pulmonary shunts.

○ *What are the patency rates of IMA and GSV cardiac bypass grafts?*

IMA - 95% 20 year patency; GSV - 80% five year patency.

○ **What patients have a moderate risk for developing endocarditis?**

Those with acquired valvular dysfunction, hypertrophic cardiomyopathy and uncorrected congenital heart defects.

○ **What is the most common organism associated with endocarditis?**

Streptococcus viridans.

○ **Fungi cause what percentage of prosthetic valve associated infective endocarditis?**

15%.

○ **What indicates severe disease in previously asymptomatic congenital aortic stenosis?**

Valvular calcifications.

○ **What is the prognosis for patients with a complete atrioventricular canal?**

Cardiac enlargement and severe cardiac failure in the first few years of life with a mortality rate of 5 to 15%.

○ *What concomitant cardiac defect is required for survival for patients with total anomalous pulmonary venous drainage?*

A patent atrial septal defect (ASD).

○ **T/F: Partial anomalous pulmonary venous drainage usually arises from the right lung.**

True.

○ **Where do left anomalous pulmonary veins usually enter the systemic circulation?**

Through a persistent left subclavian vein.

○ **What is the palliative treatment for infants with total anomalous venous drainage until definitive surgical correction can be performed?**

Balloon septoplasty.

○ **What is the appropriate treatment for patients with infective endocarditis?**

Intravenous antibiotics for 3 to 6 weeks and heparin/coumadin. Close follow-up is necessary and the patient should have a series of 2 separate negative blood cultures to demonstrate resolution of the condition.

○ **What ECG changes are associated with pericarditis?**

ST elevation in all leads except V1 and VR. PR segment depression may also be present.

○ **What is the treatment for acute pericarditis?**

Treatment of the underlying problem and anti-inflammatory agents. Steroids and narcotic analgesics may be required.

○ **Postpericardiotomy syndrome occurs in what percentage of patients who have undergone pericardiotomy?**

10 to 30%.

○ **What are the clinical manifestations of the postpericardiotomy syndrome?**

Fever, pericarditis, pleuritis and a pericardial friction rub.

○ **What signs and symptoms are associated with myocardial abscesses?**

Low-grade fevers, chills, leukocytosis, conduction system abnormalities, nonspecific ECG changes and signs and symptoms of acute MI.

○ **What is the definitive treatment for a patient with an infected myxoma?**

Surgical excision.

○ **What is the risk of infection of a transvenous pacemaker in the first 3 years after insertion?**

1 to 6%.

○ **What risk factors are associated with pacemaker infections?**

Diabetes, malignancy, skin disorders, malnutrition, anticoagulants, steroids and immunosuppressive medications.

○ **What complications are associated with pacemaker insertion?**

Post-insertion hematoma, seroma and infection.

○ **What complications are associated with infected endovascular leads?**

Valvular endocarditis, infected mural thrombi, localized abscesses and electrode perforation.

○ **What organism is most commonly associated with late infections following pacemaker insertion?**

Staphylococcus epidermidis.

○ **What is the clinical presentation of a prosthetic vascular graft infection?**

Erythema, skin breakdown and purulent drainage.

○ **What is the treatment for prosthetic vascular graft infections?**

Removal of the graft and debridement of the surrounding tissue. Extra-anatomic bypass or amputation may be required.

○ *What are the most important risk factors for line sepsis?*

In-line devices, intravenous drugs and solutions, number of lumens, number of times each lumen is handled and catheter placement.

❍ **What electrolyte abnormalities can precipitate torsades de point?**

Low potassium, magnesium, or calcium.

❍ **When should a patient quit smoking to receive the most beneficial effect prior to undergoing thoracic surgery?**

2 to 3 months prior to surgery.

❍ **Which physiologic parameters are improved with preoperative cessation of smoking?**

Closing volume, maximum voluntary ventilation and reduction in sputum production.

❍ **What is the most common type of VSD?**

Membranous septum defects.

❍ **What is the preferred approach for repair of most VSDs?**

Transatrial.

❍ *What should the post-lung resection FEV1 be prior to extubation?*

Greater than 800 ml.

❍ **What are the absolute indications for one long ventilation (OLV)?**

Protection of a healthy lung from a contaminated lung due to infection or massive hemoptysis, lavage of one lung, fistulas, surgical opening of major airways, disruption of bronchial system or unilateral cyst or bullae.

❍ **What is the most common congenital aortic arch anomaly?**

Double aortic arch.

❍ **What is the most common complication associated with mediastinoscopy?**

Hemorrhage.

❍ **What other common complications are associated with mediastenoscopy?**

Pneumothorax, recurrent nerve injury and obstruction of the innominate artery.

❍ **What are methods for lung separation?**

Bronchial blocker, endobronchial intubation and double-lumen endobronchial tube (DLT).

❍ **Which methods of lung separation can be used in children?**

Endobronchial intubation or an endobronchial blocker.

❍ **What are the disadvantages of a bronchial blocker?**

It is difficult to place, easy to obstruct the upper lobes and it moves easily.

O   **How can you aid blind placement of DLTs?**

By confirming the position with a fiberoptic bronchoscope, direct visualization by the surgeon once the chest is open or on chest x-ray.

O   **Why is a left-sided DLT more commonly used than a right-sided DLT?**

The distance of the right upper lobe bronchus and right mainstem bronchus is 2.1 cm in females and 2.3 cm in males. The distance of the left upper lobe bronchus and the left mainstem bronchus is 5 cm in females and 5.3 cm in males. Thus, it is easier to obstruct the right upper lobe.

O   **What serious complications could occur with malposition of a DLT?**

Complete obstruction of the trachea and air trapping with resulting barotrauma and cardiac arrest, tracheal or bronchial tears, compression or displacement of a mediastinal mass and possible rupture of a thoracic aneurysm.

O   **What complications are associated with high inspired oxygen?**

Oxygen toxicity and absorption (denitrogenation) atelectasis.

O   **What tidal volume and respiratory rate should be used with a DLT?**

The tidal volume should be between 10 and 12 ml/kg and the respiratory rate should be adjusted to keep the PaCO2 near 40 mm Hg.

O   **What should the peak inspiratory pressure be after lobectomy, pneumonectomy or lung transplant?**

Less than 30 mm Hg.

O   **What are the possible complications of excessive peak inspiratory pressure?**

Injury to the bronchial stump or suture line.

O   **What are the most common causes of increasing peak airway pressures with OLV?**

Malposition, kinking, obstruction or dislocation of the endotracheal tube (ETT) from surgical manipulation and secretions or debris in the ETT.

O   **What is the most common cause of arrythmias and hypotension during thoracic operations?**

Pericardial manipulation.

O   **What is hypoxic pulmonary vasoconstriction (HPV)?**

It is the pulmonary response to hypoxemia (i.e., if there is an area in the lung that is adequately oxygenated, the pulmonary vasculature will vasoconstrict in that area to divert blood to a more oxygenated area).

O   **What effects are seen with surgical stimulation of lung tissue?**

Release of prostaglandin and endothelium-derived relaxing factor, resulting in vasodilatation and increased blood flow, which increases V/Q mismatch.

O   **What is the normal shunt fraction?**

10%.

○   **What is the pathophysiology of Eisenmenger's syndrome?**

Pulmonary vascular resistance (PVR) increasing to levels greater than systemic vascular resistance (SVR) resulting in reversal of the original left-to-right shunt and cyanosis.

○   **What is the main contraindication to surgical closure of a PDA?**

Cyanosis.

○   **What is the most frequently used palliative procedure for patients with tetralogy of Fallot?**

A subclavian artery-to-pulmonary artery (Blalock-Taussis) shunt.

○   **What is the treatment of choice for patients with transposition of the great vessels?**

The arterial switch procedure.

○   **Which congenital heart defect is associated with the presence of an abnormal chamber superior and posterior to the left atrium?**

Cor triatriatum.

○   **How is cardiac involvement accessed preoperatively in a patient with a mediastinal mass?**

 CT and upright and supine echocardiography.

○   **What are the preoperative concerns for patients with myasthenia gravis (MG)?**

Possible drug interactions, history of steroid use, respiratory disease or bulbar involvement.

○   **What are the predictors of postoperative ventilatory difficulties after transsternal thymectomy for patients with MG?**

Duration of disease greater than 6 years, history of chronic respiratory disease not related to MG, pyridostigimine dosage greater than 750 mg/day and preoperative vital capacity less than 2.9 liters.

○   **A 24 year old male with a gunshot wound to the right chest is hemodynamically unstable. The entrance wound is in the second intercostal space, 1 cm lateral to the sternal border. Aortography reveals an injury of the distal innominate artery. What is the most appropriate surgical approach?**

Median sternotomy with supraclavicular extension.

○   **What patients have improved longevity with coronary artery bypass grafts (CABG)?**

Those with unstable angina, left main coronary artery disease (CAD) and those with 1-, 2- or 3-vessel disease.

○   **What is the main contraindication to CABG?**

Refractory CHF with pulmonary hypertension.

○   **What is the mortality rate of patients undergoing CABG?**

Approximately 2%.

○   **What percentage of patients have fewer episodes of angina following CABG?**

90%. Complete resolution is seen in about two-thirds of patients.

O   **What is the appropriate therapy for patients with refractory angina?**

Emergent percutaneous transluminal coronary angioplasty (PTCA) or CABG.

O   **A 51 year old male underwent CABG 5 hours ago and suddenly becomes hypotensive with a cardiac index (CI) of 1.5 l/min, central venous pressure (CVP) of 20 mm Hg, left atrial pressure of 24 mm Hg and has significantly increased drainage from his mediastinal thoracostomy tube. What is the treatment of choice?**

Immediate mediastinal re-exploration.

O   **T/F: Patients with refractory angina and left main CAD should be treated with PTCA.**

False.

O   **What are the most common causes of aortic stensosis in adults?**

Rheumatic fever or a long bicuspid valve.

O   **What are the indications for valve replacement in patients with aortic stenosis?**

Symptomatic patients, systolic pressure gradient greater than 50 mm Hg, valvular cross-sectional area less than 1 cm^2 and serial x-ray evidence of rapid cardiac enlargement.

O   **What are the typical symptoms of anterior circulation cerebrovascular ischemia?**

Aphasia, contralateral weakness or sensory change in the upper or lower extremities and contralateral facial droop.

O   **What clinical symptoms are most typical of vertebrobasilar ischemia?**

Diplopia, dizziness, syncope, dysarthria, ataxia and bilateral extremity sensory change or weakness.

O   **What is the mortality rate for patients requiring permanent anticoagulation therapy?**

1 to 2% per year.

O   *Following a high-speed motor vehicle accident (MVA), evaluation reveals a widened mediastinum. What is the pathophysiology of the probable injury?*

The ligamentum arteriosum tethers the under surface of the aortic arch to the proximal left main pulmonary artery, at a point just distal to the left subclavian artery. Sudden deceleration causes shearing between the mobile aortic arch and the immobile descending aorta, resulting in aortic disruption.

O   *Following an MVA where the patient was wearing a shoulder strap, the only notable physical findings are left neck tenderness with mild ecchymosis and a brief episode of aphasia reported by rescue workers at the scene. A duplex carotid Doppler study reveals a small intimal flap in the distal common carotid artery. What is the most appropriate management of this patient?*

Surgical repair.

O   **What are the characteristics of fibromuscular dysplasia in the carotid artery?**

Alternating short intervals of dilation and stenotic fibromuscular thickenings, turbulence with thromboembolic events, transient ischemic attacks, stroke and intracranial aneurysms.

❍   **What are the boundaries for classification and management of penetrating neck injuries?**

Zone I extends from the clavicle to the cricoid cartilage, zone II extends from the cricoid cartilage to the angle of the mandible and zone III extends from the angle of the mandible to the base of the skull.

❍   **What are the typical features of Takayasu's arteritis?**

Early symptoms include fever, myalgias, arthralgias, weight loss and pain over inflamed vessels. Late symptoms are referable to occlusive changes and include transient ischemic attacks, strokes, arm fatigue, leg claudication and angina.

❍   **What are the arteriographic findings of Takayasu's disease?**

Segmental dilatations, stenoses and occlusions.

❍   **What is the treatment for patients with Takayasu's disease?**

Surgery is required for the treatment of aneurysmal and stenotic lesions with failure of medical management.

❍   **What are the typical features of giant cell (temporal) arteritis?**

A flu-like prodrome with fever, malaise, weight loss, scalp tenderness, headache and myalgias. Pain over the temporal or occipital arteries, jaw claudication and eye symptoms follow.

❍   **What is the etiology of transient monocular blindness (amaurosis fugax) in patients with temporal arteritis?**

Occlusion of the terminal retinal arterioles from atherosclerotic emboli arising from the carotid bifurcation.

❍   **What rheumatologic condition is frequently associated with temporal arteritis?**

Polymyalgia rheumatica.

❍   **What is the appropriate management of Paget-Schroetter syndrome?**

Heparinization, direct infusion thrombolysis, thoracic outlet decompression and percutaneous angioplasty if residual venous stenosis exists. Venoplasty is occasionally required.

❍   **What is the appropriate management for a neonate with hypoplastic left heart syndrome (HPHS)?**

Prostagandin infusion.

❍   **What is the most appropriate exposure for a penetrating injury to the mid subclavian artery?**

Subperiosteal or complete removal of the medial portion of the clavicle combined with division of the anterior scalene muscle provides exposure to the middle and distal left subclavian artery and all three portions of the right subclavian artery.

❍   **What are the signs and symptoms of the subclavian steal syndrome?**

Dizziness, diplopia, ataxia and bilateral sensory or motor deficits or syncope when exercising the ipsilateral arm.

❍   **What are the indications for patch closure of a carotid endarterectomy (CEA)?**

Patients with small arteries and re-do endarterectomies for recurrent stenosis.

O   **A 67 year old male states that he had a 3-hour episode of left arm numbness and extreme weakness. The physical exam is significant for a right carotid bruit and a very subtle decrease in left grip strength. What is the appropriate management?**

A head CT scan without contrast, ECG, echocardiography and a carotid duplex study. Increasingly, experienced vascular surgeons proceed to endarterectomy without angiography in appropriate clinical situations.

O   **Which artery must frequently be divided to gain exposure to the hypoglossal nerve during CEA?**

The artery to the sternocleidomastoid muscle.

O   **What are the branches of the external carotid artery?**

In order from proximal to distal, the superior thyroid, ascending pharyngeal, lingual, facial, occipital, posterior auricular, internal maxillary and temporal arteries.

O   **What conditions are associated with aortic dissection?**

Connective tissue disorders such as Marfan's and Ehlers-Danlos syndromes, congenital heart lesions (e.g., bicuspid aortic valve and coarctation) and uncontrolled hypertension.

O   **What is the DeBakey system of aortic dissection classification?**

Type 1 involves the ascending aorta, aortic arch and thoracoabdominal aorta. Type 2 dissections have a false channel limited to the ascending aorta. Type 3 dissections are divided into 3a (beginning distal to the left subclavian artery and terminating above the diaphragm) and 3b (beginning distal to the left subclavian artery and extending into the abdominal aorta).

O   **What is the initial mainstay of medical therapy in all types of acute aortic dissection?**

Intensive continuous monitoring. Cardiac output and blood pressure must be promptly reduced to as low a level as possible while still maintaining end-organ-perfusion. Sodium nitroprusside is the first line antihypertensive agent (infused at 1 to 2 mcg/kg/min to maintain systolic blood pressure at 90 to 100 mm Hg or lower, if needed for pain control). Simultaneous intravenous beta blockade with esmolol is administered to prevent tachycardia and maintain a heart rate less than 70.

O   **During CEA, what hemodynamic changes may occur with manipulation of the carotid bulb?**

Bradycardia and hypotension.

O   *What is the treatment for these hemodynamic changes?*

Injection of 1 or 2 cc of 1% plain lidocaine into the carotid bulb periadventitial tissue. Systemic atropine may be considered for persistent intraoperative bradycardia. Postoperative bradycardia may be treated with judicious administration of atropine in the symptomatic patient. Occasionally, low dose infusion of Neo-Synephrine is needed to maintain an appropriate mean arterial pressure.

O   **With respect to CEA, what intraoperative measures minimize the risk of perioperative stroke?**

Smooth induction of anesthesia, avoidance of hemodynamic instability and resultant low cerebral blood flow, meticulous dissection of the carotid artery with minimal manipulation, selective shunting, appropriate flushing and back-bleeding of the arteries, anticoagulation and meticulous closure.

O   **What is the Stanford classification of aortic dissection?**

Stanford type A dissection involves the ascending aorta. Type B dissection begins distal to the origin of the left subclavian artery.

O **What are the criteria for surgical management of aortic dissection?**

All acute type A dissections should be treated with emergent operation including replacement or repair of the ascending aorta, aortic root and aortic valve. Acute type B dissections are treated with early surgical intervention if visceral or extremity arterial origins are compromised.

O **What are the 3 types of recurrent carotid stenosis?**

Myointimal hyperplasia, recurrent atherosclerotic lesions and residual plaque left from the primary operation.

O **Other than arch aortography, what diagnostic tests may be helpful in ruling out traumatic aortic disruption?**

Transesophageal echocardiography and spiral CT scan of the chest.

O **Following left carotid-subclavian bypass, a patient developed a large amount of serous drainage from the wound. What is the most likely diagnosis?**

Injury to the thoracic duct.

O **What is the most common benign cardiac tumor?**

Myxoma.

O **What is the most common cardiac tumor in infancy?**

Rhabdomyoma.

O **What organisms are most frequently implicated in endocarditis in intravenous drug abusers?**

Gram negative and fungal organisms.

O **What is the most important regulator of coronary blood flow?**

Adenosine.

O **What percentage of premature infants have successful closure of a PDA with indomethacin?**

50%.

O **What are the relative contraindications to the use of indomethacin for neonates with PDA?**

Intracranial hemorrhage, nephritis and enterocolitis.

O **What is the treatment of choice for patients with asymptomatic aortic stenosis?**

Valvulotomy.

O **What is the incidence of recurrent stenosis after valvulotomy?**

20 to 30%.

O **What is the definition of a reversible ischemic neurologic deficit (RIND)?**

Ischemic or embolic cerebral infarction resulting in neurologic deficits that last longer than 24 hours but resolve within 3 weeks.

O   **What is the etiology of idiopathic hypertrophic subaortic stenosis (IHSS)?**

A hypertrophic myopathy of the left ventricular outflow tract.

O   **In performing repair of an ASD, there is poor decompression of the right heart despite achieving good bypass with bicaval cannulation. What is the most likely diagnosis?**

A persistent left superior vena cava.

O   *A 6 month old presents with sweating and irritability while feeding. Chest x-ray demonstrates a markedly enlarged cardiac silhouette and echocardiogram reveals a dilated, poorly contractile left ventricle with moderate to severe mitral regurgitation. What is the most likely diagnosis?*

Anomalous origin of the left coronary artery from the pulmonary artery.

O   **T/F: Anomalous left coronary artery from the pulmonary artery is best treated by reimplantation of the coronary artery into the aorta.**

True.

O   **What congenital heart lesion is the most common cause of cyanosis presenting in the newborn period?**

Transposition of the great vessels.

O   **What complications are associated with surgical repair of coarctation of the aorta?**

Paraplegia and postoperative hypertension.

O   **An eight year old child presents with cyanosis but is otherwise asymptomatic. Cardiac catheterization reveals the following:**

Site	Pressure (mm Hg)	Oxygen saturation
Superior vena cava	5	61%
Right atrium	5	62%
Right ventricle	100/5	64%
Pulmonary artery	100/60	67%
Left atrium	8	98%
Left ventricle	100/8	89%
Aorta	100/70	82%

What is the most likely diagnosis?

VSD with high pulmonary vascular resistance (Eisenmenger's syndrome).

O   **What are the indications for ventricular aneurysm resection?**

CHF, recurrent malignant ventricular arrhythmias, angina pectoris and peripheral embolization.

O   **What is the etiology of the typical heart murmur seen in patients with an ASD?**

Flow across the pulmonic valve.

O   **What is involved in the repair of an AV canal defect?**

Placing a patch to close the VSD, another patch to close the atrial septal defect and division and resuspension of the common AV valve into a left sided (corresponding to the mitral valve) and right sided (corresponding to the tricuspid valve) component.

O   **A 6 month old with a VSD undergoes cardiac catheterization with the following findings:**

Sitez	Pressure (mm Hg)	Oxygen saturation
Superior vena cava	5	65%
Right atrium	5	66%
Right ventricle	70/5	75%
Pulmonary artery	65/20	90%
Left atrium	7	98%
Left ventricle	75/7	98%
Aorta	75/40	98%

What is the degree of left to right shunt?

4:1. (SaO2 - SvO2) / (SpvO2 - SpaO2), where SaO2 is the systemic arterial oxygen saturation (aorta), SvO2 is the mixed venous oxygen saturation (superior vena cava), SpvO2 is the oxygen saturation in the pulmonary veins (left atrium) and SpaO2 is the oxygen saturation in the pulmonary artery.

O   **A 4 day old infant presents with shock and severe acidosis. Echocardiogram demonstrates an interrupted aortic arch, type B. What is the next step in management?**

Continuous infusion of prostaglandin E1.

O   **What disorder is likely to accompany the patient in the question above?**

DiGeorge syndrome (thymic aplasia).

O   **A 9 month old child has progressive cyanosis but is otherwise asymptomatic. Echocardiogram demonstrates tetralogy of Fallot. Complete repair is contemplated and cardiac catheterization is proposed. What is the most important information to be obtained from the catheterization?**

The coronary artery anatomy.

O   **What are the clinical characteristics of chronic constrictive pericarditis?**

Progressive edema, ascites, hepatomegaly and exertional dyspnea.

O   **What is the treatment of choice for patients with constrictive pericarditis?**

Pericardiectomy.

O   **At what age should the arterial switch procedure be performed for patients with transposition of the great vessels?**

Usually at 1 to 2 weeks of age.

O   **Following dacron patch repair of a paramembranous VSD, a patient develops complete heart block. What is the most appropriate next step?**

Epicardial pacing.

O   **What is the most likely location of the conduction system in the above patient?**

Along the posteroinferior border of paramembranous VSD.

O   **What are the indications for PTCA?**

Acute evolving MI, critical coronary stenosis, stenotic vein bypass grafts, intraoperative dilatation of distal segmental lesions and distal bypass grafts and patients with 1- or 2-vessel disease.

O   **What is the embryological origin of an ostium secundum ASD?**

A deficiency of the septum primum.

O   **What is the appropriate treatment for critical aortic stenosis diagnosed in the neonate?**

Balloon valvulotomy.

O   **What auscultatory finding is associated with aortic insufficiency?**

A decrescendo diastolic murmur. A systolic ejection murmur may also be heard.

O   **What is the most common primary malignant cardiac neoplasm?**
Sarcoma.

O   *What are the indication for use of an intra-arterial balloon pump (IABP)?*

Cardiac failure after cardiopulmonary bypass, refractory unstable angina, preoperative therapy for septal defects, arrhythmias, ventricular aneurysms and cardiogenic shock.

O   **An 8 year old male is brought to the ER by his mother who states that he has been having chest pain. Physical exam reveals a systolic ejection murmur and a precordial thrill. Chest x-ray is normal. What is the treatment of choice?**

Aortic valve replacement.

❍ **A 1 week old female is brought to the ER by her parents because she is "turning blue." The infant is clearly cyanotic and her stat chest x-ray reveals an egg-shaped heart. What test will confirm your diagnosis?**

Echocardiography.

❍ **A 45 year old female presents with angina and has a positive stress test. What is the next step in management?**

Angiography.

❍ **T/F: The operative mortality for CABG is higher in women than in men.**

True.

❍ **What is the most common complication of ascending thoracic aorta aneurysms?**

Aortic valve insufficiency.

VASCULAR SURGERY PEARLS

I don't want to achieve immortality through my work.
I want to achieve it through not dying.
Woody Allen

○ **What are the cardiovascular variables associated with aortic cross clamping at the infrarenal level?**

Minimal changes. There is a 2% increase in mean arterial pressure (MAP), no change in the left ventricular end-diastolic pressure (LVEDP) and a reduction in the ejection fraction (EF) of 3%. Supra-celiac clamping however, results in significant increased LVEDP and subsequent left heart strain.

○ **What are the determinants of cerebral blood flow during carotid endarterectomy (CEA)?**

Partial pressure of arterial CO_2 and O_2 ($PaCO_2$ and PaO_2), arterial blood pressure, autoregulation, venous blood pressure, anesthetic drugs, metabolic factors (i.e., seizures and shivering) and pain.

○ **How is the stump pressure used in CEA?**

It is dependent upon extracranial collateral flow, systemic pressure and cerebrovascular resistance. Pressures of 40-50 mm Hg are thought to indicate adequate flow. However, the correlation between EEGs and stump pressure is less than good, since flow does not necessarily indicate adequate perfusion.

○ **What is the most common cause of late failure of reversed saphenous vein grafts?**

Atherosclerosis.

○ **What is the appropriate treatment for superficial thrombophlebitis without evidence of clot extension into the deep venous system?**

Local heat, NSAIDs and continued ambulation.

○ **What is the treatment of choice for superficial thrombophlebitis if the thrombus propagates towards the deep system?**

Short or long saphenous vein ligation. Excision of the involved vein is indicated in patients with persistence of symptoms despite medical therapy and recurrent episodes of thrombophlebitis.

○ **What is the mortality rate for ruptured abdominal aortic aneurysms (AAA) who arrive at the hospital alive?**

30 to 50%.

○ **What are the drawbacks of contrast venography in the diagnosis of deep vein thrombosis (DVT)?**

It is a costly, time consuming and painful study with a 10% interobserver diagnostic disagreement. In addition to complications related to the contrast medium, mild and major idiosyncratic reactions cause nephrotoxicity and provide little physiologic information. Finally, it is difficult to demonstrate the presence of thrombus in muscle sinusoids, the profunda femoris or internal iliac veins.

❍   **What are the normal lower extremity venous Doppler flow patterns?**

A venous Doppler signal is low pitched, containing a wide spectrum of frequencies. (It sounds like a windstorm.) In supine subjects, the flow in the legs is phasic with respiration. With abdominal breathing, it increases with expiration and decreases with inspiration.

❍   **T/F: Compliance of synthetic arterial grafts is greater than that of the normal arterial system.**

False.

❍   **T/F: Intravenous pyelography (IVP) is the diagnostic test of choice for renovascular hypertension.**

False, angiography is the gold standard diagnostic tool.

❍   **What is the most common site for atherosclerotic occlusion in the lower extremities?**

The distal superficial femoral artery.

❍   *What is the most common etiologic factor involved in ascending aortic aneurysms?*

Cystic medial necrosis.

❍   **What is the expected ankle-brachial index (ABI) in patients with intermittent claudication?**

Between 1.0 and 0.5.

❍   **What are the Doppler signs of acute DVT?**

Absence of flow in a vein segment, continuous (nonphasic) flow distal to an obstruction, lack of augmentation proximal to an obstruction and increased flow in the superficial veins.

❍   **Repair of which type of aneurysm is associated with the highest operative mortality rate?**

Transverse aortic arch aneurysms.

❍   **What are the limitations of using Doppler as opposed to duplex ultrasound for the diagnosis of acute DVT?**

Poor detection of tibial vein thromboses, inability to differentiate acute from chronic venous obstructive disease and inability to detect nonocclusive thrombi.

❍   **How accurate is a ventilation/perfusion (V/Q) scan in diagnosis of acute pulmonary embolus (PE)?**

Pulmonary angiography has shown that in a patient with a high probability V/Q scan, the incidence of PE is 87%. With an intermediate probability reading, the incidence is 30% and with a low probability reading, the incidence is 14%.

❍   **What are the indications for an emergency pulmonary embolectomy?**

Persistent refractory hypotension despite maximal resuscitation in a patient with a documented acute, massive PE.

❍   **What is the natural history of valvular reflux after an acute DVT?**

Valvular reflux develops progressively from the time of acute DVT.

❍ *What is the appropriate treatment for a 30 year old male with an asymptomatic 3 cm splenic artery aneurysm?*

Surgical repair of the aneurysm.

❍ *What is the treatment of choice for acute arterial embolus to the lower extremity?*

Immediate heparization. Surgical embolectomy or intra-arterial thrombolytic therapy with angioget. Must watch for reperfusion injury associated compartment syndrome and rhabdomyolysis.

❍ **What is the diagnostic test of choice for venous or arterial disease?**

Doppler ultrasonography with B-mode ultrasonography.

❍ **What is the contraindication to thromboendarterectomy?**

Concomitant aneurysmal disease.

❍ **What is the initial pathophysiologic event in the development of atherosclerosis?**

Platelet adherence.

❍ **What is the appropriate treatment for subclavian steal syndrome?**

Carotid-subclavian or axilloaxillary bypass or angioplasty and stenting of the subclavian artery.

❍ **What is the treatment of choice for patients with Leriche syndrome?**

Aortoiliac-bifemoral bypass or iliac angioplasty and stenting if short segment ammenanble lesions.

❍ **What are the prerequisites for success of a cross-femoral venous bypass for relief of symptoms due to a chronically occluded iliac vein?**

Patency of the contralateral iliofemoral and caval runoff, presence of a supine resting pressure gradient in excess of 4 to 5 mm Hg between the femoral veins in the involved and contralateral limbs and a good quality contralateral saphenous vein.

❍ *What is the appropriate management of reperfusion injury following vascular repair?*

Serum electrolyte evaluation and intravenous administration of sodium bicarbonate and mannitol. PRN fasciotomy.

❍ **What is Milroy's disease?**

Familial lymphedema that is present at birth or is noticed soon thereafter.

❍ **What is the preferred replacement material for pediatric renal artery reconstruction?**

Arterial autograft.

❍ **T/F: Patients with a carotid bruit have an increased risk of stroke during abdominal surgery.**

False.

❍ **What is the most common functional type of primary lymphedema?**

Distal lymphatic obliteration.

❍   **What is the Charles' procedure for treatment of lymphedema?**

Excision of the skin and subcutaneous tissues in the involved extremity and closure of the resulting defect with a skin graft.

❍   **What factors are predictive of healing following amputation?**

A segmental arterial pressure of 50 mm Hg at the level of planned amputation and a TcPO2 greater than 50 Torr for the skin flap.

❍   **What is the appropriate management of chronic lymphedema?**

Elevation of the legs, compression stockings when ambulating, periodic compression pumps for severe cases and manual lymph drainage.

❍   **What is the treatment of choice for a patient with unilateral ilioaortic occlusion and an intraabdominal infection?**

Femorofemoral crossover graft.

❍   **T/F: Impedance plethysmography (IPG) is less accurate than duplex scanning for detection of chronic DVT.**

True.

❍   **What are the roles of the carotid body and sinus respectively?**

Body (@bifurcation) detects increased BP and triggers bradycardia and BP fall. Sinus (along internal carotid) is a chemoreceptor which detects increased CO2/H+ and triggers tachycardia.

❍   **What is the most common manifestation of chemodactomas?**

A painless neck mass.

❍   **What is the most common cause of arterial mycotic aneurysms?**

Use of prosthetic graft material.

❍   *What is the appropriate treatment for a patient with symptomatic carotid stenosis on the right and asymptomatic 50% stenosis on the left?*

CEA on the symptomatic side only.

❍   *What are the characteristic symptoms of vertebral basilar ischemia?*

Diplopia, dysarthria, vertigo and tinnitus.

❍   **Who is likely to benefit from the surgical treatment of chronic lymphedema of the lower extremity?**

Patients with restricted movement and functional impairment due to gross enlargement of the extremity and those who experience frequent episodes of lymphangitis.

❍   **T/F: Long-term patency of above-knee femoropopliteal bypass with polytetrafluoroethylene (PTFE) has comparable patency rates with those of venous autografts.**

False.

❍   **What are the indications for tibioperoneal bypass grafts?**

Gangrene of the forefoot, rest pain, necrotizing infection or a nonhealing wound.

❍   **What are the alternatives to intraarterial contrast angiography?**

Duplex examination, intraarterial ultrasound, CT angiography, MRA and angioscopy.

❍   **How is carotid arterial stenosis measured from an arteriogram?**

By comparing the diameter of the stenotic area with the diameter of the nondiseased distal internal carotid artery. This ratio is subtracted from one and expresses the percentage of diameter reduction.

❍   *What is the success rate of angioplasty for the following anatomic sites: iliac, femoral, popliteal and tibial?*

At 5 years, iliac angioplasty with stenting has a 90% success rate, 60% without a stent. Femoropopliteal success rates approximate 30% at 5 years and tibial lesions are considerably lower.

❍   **What are the characteristics of fibromuscular dysplasia (FMD)?**

Eccentric stenoses with intervening areas of dilatation.

❍   *What is the major concern in a patient who develops bloody diarrhea following AAA repair?*

Ischemic colitis secondary to loss of the IMA with inadequate collateral circulation.

❍   **What is the leading cause of late death after aortic reconstruction?**

CAD.

❍   **How much of the small intestine can be resected without creating a nutritional cripple?**

Up to 70%.

❍   *Blunt carotid injury is best managed how?*

Anticoagulation.

❍   **What is the treatment of choice for patients with FMD?**

Percutaneous transluminal angioplasty (PTA) if ammenable, or renal artery bypass.

❍   **What type of aortic aneurysm is associated with Marfan's syndrome?**

Type A.

❍   *What causes the blood pressure fluctuation commonly seen after carotid surgery?*

Manipulation of the carotid body.

❍   *What is the appropriate management for a 23 year old male smoker who presents with symptoms of upper extremity ischemia?*

Patients with Buerger's disease are encouraged to quit smoking and are managed with analgesics.

○   *What is the treatment of choice for patients with superior vena cava (SVC) syndrome caused by malignancy?*

Radiation therapy.

○   *What are the causes of reduced urine output after aortic reconstructive procedures?*

Inadequate circulating blood volume, low cardiac output (CO), renal ischemia, acute tubular necrosis (ATN) and a kinked or clogged Foley catheter.

○   **What are the benefits of CEA versus antiplatelet agents in symptomatic carotid disease?**

CEA produces a 7-fold reduction in the long-term risk of stroke.

○   *There are two landmark studies in vascular surgery, which give strong implications for CEA vs medical management of carotid disease. What are these studies and what are the important statistics for each?*

ACAS- Asymptomatic pts with > 60% stenosis who underwent CEA there is a 5 yr reduction in CVA rate of 11% to 5%.

NASCET- Symtomatic pts with > 70% stenosis CEA reduces 2 year CVA rate
From 26% to 9%.

○   **A popliteal aneurysm is palpated in your pt. What are the chances he has another aneurysm?**

50% are bilateral and 1/3 have a AAA.

○   *T/F: Conservative management is acceptable for non symptomatic popliteal aneurysm 2.1 cm in size?*

False. These have a high risk of emboli and thrombus, therefore operation by exclusion and bypass is standard of care. 2 cm is the threshold for repair.

○   **What are some of the risk factors associated with AAA increase in size?**

HTN, COPD, smoking.

○   **What are the 5 year risk of rupture of AAA based on size?**

5 cm- 20%.
>7 cm- 95%.

○   *What percentage of patients initially experience endoleak post endovascular AAA repair?*

50%, these are typically observed for up to a year because of spontaneous cessation and low rupture rate if the aneurysm sac is not rapidly expanding.

○   **What is dysphagia lusoria?**

Dysphagia secondary to an aberrant right subclavian artery traveling between the esophagus and the trachea. Can be diagnosed by pulsations seen on EGD.

○   **What is the most common visceral aneurysm?**

Splenic artery aneurysm.

○   **What are the indications for surgery for splenic aneurysm?**

>2 cm, female of child bearing age or planning pregnancy, any Symptomatic pt.

O   **What is the recurrence rate of ipsilateral internal carotid stenosis following CEA?**

10 to 15%.

O   *The initial treatment of Takayasu's arteritis is?*

Steroid therapy.

O   **What is the most common cause of renovascular hypertension?**

Atherosclerosis.

O   **What is the earliest objective measurement reflecting compartment syndrome?**

Compartment pressure greater than 40 mm Hg.

O   **What is the characteristic gross appearance of an inflammatory AAA?**

An intense, thick, white fibroplastic reaction with adherence to the third and fourth portions of the duodenum and the inferior vena cava (IVC).

O   **What is the most common cause of cerebral ischemia?**

Arterioarterial emboli.

O   **What is the appropriate treatment for infected prosthetic grafts?**

Antibiotics, removal of the prosthesis and re-establishment of vascular continuity.

O   **What percentage of patients with traumatic thoracic aortic aneurysms survive long enough for a false aneurysm to develop?**

2%.

O   *What are the indications for an IVC filter?*

PE despite theraputic anticoagulation; DVT in a patient with firm contra-indication to anticoagulation.

O   **What should be done for a patient who awakens with a new ipsilateral neurologic deficit following CEA?**

Immediate bedside duplex, angiogram and/or re-exploration.

O   *Which is the most common CN injured in CEA?*

Vagus.

O   **A young women presents to your office and has HTN and carries the diagnosis of Fibromuscular dysplasia. Upon angiogram you see the lesion is in the right renal artery.   (Most common location). What are the surgical treatment options?**

Angioplasty or bypass.

O   **What noninvasive tests are used to assess the severity of claudication?**

Resting segmental pressures and pulse-volume recordings may demonstrate occlusive disease. A graded-treadmill protocol will quantify the distance the patient can walk and demonstrate the typical pressure drop at the ankle following exercise.

○   **Does TIPS procedure increase the rate of encephalopathy?**

Yes, it approaches 25%.

○   **What is Pagett-Schroetter syndrome?**

Axillosubclavian venous thrombosis secondary to thoracic outlet syndrome.

○   ***The best method to evaluate whether a toe amputation in a diabetic patient will heal is?***

Measurement of toe pressures.

○   **What is the appropriate treatment for patients with post-phlebitic syndrome?**

Compression of the lower extremity with stockings of a prescribed pressure, usually 20 to 40 mm Hg. For patients with ulcerations, medicated wraps, such as the Una boot, are used until healing occurs. For those who do not heal, endoscopic ligation of perforating veins has become an important new technique to reduce local venous pressure.

○   ***Name some features of Buerger's disease.***

Smokers, involvement of vessels distal to the elbow and knee joints, no co-existing connective tissue disease, 80% male, smoking cessation initial treatment in absence of gangrene, corkscrew collaterals on angiography.

○   ***What is the natural history of untreated popliteal artery aneurysms?***

It tends to thrombose acutely or be a source for distal emboli and cause limb-threatening ischemia.

○   ***What is the relationship of a popliteal aneurysm to an AAA?***

30-40% of patients with a unilateral popliteal aneurysm may have an AAA; 50% have a contralateral popliteal aneurysm.

○   ***3 days after a AAA repair your pt has bloody diarrhea. What test should you perform?***

Initial hb, then follow with sigmoidoscopy to evaluate for ischemic colon. This occurs secondary to loss of IMA.

○   ***Your pt complains of claudication what initial surgery is most beneficial?***

None. Life style modification such as exercise, cessation smoking are the initial treatment.

○   ***What is the mechanism of renovascular hypertension?***

The renal juxtaglomerular apparatus (JGA), through the renin-angiotensin system, seeks to maintain a normal arterial pressure at the JGA. Stenotic arterial lesions proximal to the kidney cause the JGA to secrete renin, which through the angiotensin cascade, raises the central pressure above normal and, therefore, the pressure at the JGA (beyond the stenosis) rises towards normal.

○   **What is the thoracic outlet?**

The thoracic outlet is an anatomic structure formed by the first rib, clavicle and scalene muscles through which pass the brachial plexus, subclavian artery and subclavian vein. The nerves and artery are posterior to the vein and separated by the anterior scalene muscle.

O **What is thoracic outlet syndrome?**

Anything that narrows the outlet, such as muscular hypertrophy, fibrous tissue, scar tissue or fracture callus, can impinge on one or more of the structures within the thoracic outlet and cause symptoms.

O **What is Virchow's Triad?**

Stasis, endothelial cell injury and a hypercoagulable state.

O **New onset neurologic deficit 90 minutes post CEA on the side opposite the operation should be managed how?**

Re-exploration of the ICA due to a high probability of in-situ thrombosis.

O **What patients are at increased risk for DVT?**

Those with hypercoagulable body chemistries, previous DVT, lower-extremity trauma, orthopedic surgery, major pelvic operations, immobility, acute MI, CHF, malignancies and those taking oral contraceptives, especially if they smoke.

O **What are the effective prophylactic measures for DVT?**

Coumadin, unfractionated heparin, low-molecular weight heparins, dextran, antiplatelet drugs such as aspirin or ticlid, and sequential venous compression stockings (SCDs).

O *What is Charcot foot in the diabetic patient?*

Inflammatory osteoarthropathy in the tarsal bones resulting in collapsed plantar arch.

CHEST WALL, LUNG, PLEURA AND MEDIASTINUM PEARLS

The best way to stop smoking is to carry wet matches.
Anonymous

○   **The inferior pulmonary vein of the lung lies within what structure?**

The pulmonary ligament.

○   **T/F: At the level of the carina, the pulmonary arteries lie anterior to the mainstem bronchi and posterior to the aortic arch.**

True.

○   **When performing a posterolateral thoracotomy, what chest wall muscles are usually transected?**

The latissimus dorsi and serratus anterior.

○   **What laboratory values suggest that a pleural effusion is an exudate?**

Pleural fluid/serum protein ratio greater than 0.5, pleural fluid/serum LDH ratio greater than 0.6.

○   **What is the most common etiology of a spontaneous pneumothorax?**

Rupture of a pulmonary bleb.

○   **At what level do the Vena cava, esophagus, thoracic duct, and aorta cross the diaphragm?**

Vena cava- T8.
Esophagus- T10.
Aorta+Thoracic duct- 12.

○   **What protozoa is responsible for a diffuse interstitial pneumonitis in immunocompromised patients?**

Pneumocystis carinii.

○   **What is the standard therapy for a lung abscess?**

Systemic antibiotics, bronchoscopy to remove any foreign body and to exclude endobronchial tumor or obstruction.

○   **What is the most common form of non-small cell lung cancer in the United States?**

Adenocarcinoma.

○   **What is the most common benign tumor of the lung?**

Hamartoma.

O   **What are the most common primary malignant tumors of the chest wall?**

Myeloma and chondrosarcoma.

O   **What is the most common benign tumor of the chest wall?**

Osteochondroma.

O   **Which lung neoplasm, in young to middle-aged patients, is often centrally located, usually endobronchial and may present with obstructive symptoms or hemoptysis?**

Bronchopulmonary carcinoid.

O   *Prior to Thoracotomy pfts are ordered on pts. The pts need certain FEV1's to insure good outcome after procedure. What is the prethoracotomy PFT for pneumonectomy/ lobectomy/wedge?*

Pneumonectomy- 2L.
Lobectomy- 1L.

O   **In lung cancer paraneoplastic syndromes, which lung ca is associated with increase Ca?**

Squamous cell.

O   **When is a lung Ca unresectable?**

N3- contralateral or subclavian or scalene involvement.
T4- mediastinal, heart, great vessel, esophagus, trachea, vertebaral, or effusion (midline major structures).
Resectable- chest wall, pericardium, diaphragm invasion.

O   *What preoperative arterial blood gas (ABG) values imply an increased risk of respiratory insufficiency following pulmonary resection?*

PCO2 greater than 45 Torr and PaO2 less than 50 Torr.

O   *T/F: A 60 year old male with a preoperative FEV1 of 1.8 and a pulmonary ventilation-perfusion (V/Q) scan showing 60% function from the left lung is not at increased risk of postoperative respiratory insufficiency following left pneumonectomy.*

True.

O   **T/F: A patient with a preoperative MVV of 75% predicted, a normal ABG and an FEV1 of 1.7 requires no further evaluation prior to pulmonary resection.**

False.

O   **What percentage of patients diagnosed with non-small cell lung cancer have the potential to undergo surgical resection for cure?**

30%.

O   **T/F: Mediastinal lymph nodes that appear larger than 1.0 cm in size on CT scan confer N2 (stage IIIA) disease, precluding curative resection of non-small-cell lung cancer.**

False.

○ *What tuype of tumor should one think of when pt presents with ptosis, miosis, and anhydrosis, and ulnar nerve injury findings?*

Pancost, invasion of the sympathetic chain/stellate ganglion inducing horner's syndrome.

○ **What is the treatment of choice for an isolated brain metastasis that otherwise appears to have stage I non-small cell lung cancer?**

Resection of the isolated brain metastasis followed by whole brain irradiation and resection of the primary lung tumor.

○ **What stage disease does the above patient have?**

Stage IV.

○ **What is the appropriate treatment for a superior sulcus (Pancoast) tumor?**

Radiation followed by surgical resection or a definitive dose (60 to 65 Gy) of radiation.

○ **T/F: An ipsilateral pleural effusion is a contraindication to curative resection for non-small cell lung cancer.**

False.

○ **What is the 5-year survival of patients undergoing complete resection of a stage IA (T1N0M0) non-small cell lung cancer?**

70%.

○ **T/F: Postoperative radiation therapy for non-small cell lung cancer improves patient survival.**

False. However, it has been shown to decrease the rate of local recurrence in patients with completely resected stage II and III squamous cell carcinoma of the lung.

○ **When is a pneumonectomy required for the resection of non-small cell lung cancer?**

When there is tumor invasion of the proximal mainstem bronchus or pulmonary arteries or veins in patients without other contraindications to resection.

○ **Horner's syndrome is most often associated with which intrathoracic malignancy?**

Superior sulcus (Pancoast) tumor.

○ *Does resecting thymus in myasthenia improve symptoms?*

Yes. 90% of pts improve. 10% of pts with myastenia gravis have a thymoma, however one does not need a thymoma for symptoms of MG to improve.

○ **What is the preferred technique for resection of metastases to the lung?**

Wedge resection.

○ **T/F: There is a greater survival benefit to lobectomy over segmentectomy and wedge resection in the treatment of a peripheral T1N0M0 (stage IA) non-small cell lung cancer.**

True. Lobectomy improves 5-year survival and reduces the incidence of locoregional recurrence from 15% to 5%.

O   **What is the appropriate treatment of a right upper lobe non-small cell lung cancer involving the orifice of the right upper lobe but not extending into the bronchus intermedius or involving regional lymph nodes?**

Right upper lobectomy with anastomosis of the bronchus intermedius to the mainstem bronchus.

O   *T/F: Non-small cell lung cancer that invades the parietal pleura or chest wall is not resectable for cure and should be treated with radiation.*

False.

O   **What is the preferred therapy for patients with superior vena cava syndrome caused by non-small cell lung cancer?**

Radiation therapy.

O   **Which fungus has a propensity to colonize a pre-existing pulmonary cavity?**

Aspergillus.

O   **What are the current indications for surgical resection of pulmonary tuberculosis?**

Persistent or recurrent infection despite adequate multi-drug therapy, massive or recurrent hemoptysis, inability to exclude carcinoma and bronchopleural fistula unresponsive to tube thoracostomy.

O   **What is the best initial method for localizing hemoptysis in a patient who is actively bleeding?**

Bronchoscopy.

O   *What type of bronchopulmonary sequestration has a distinct pleural investment, no communication with the tracheobronchial tree, an arterial supply derived from small systemic arteries and systemic venous drainage?*

Extralobar sequestration.; intralobar have pulmonary venous return and a bronchial attachment to the pulmonary tree.

O   **What is the initial bedside therapy for an acute bronchopleural fistula following pneumonectomy?**

Turn the patient operated side down to prevent aspiration of pleural fluid into the contralateral lung and tube thoracostomy.

O   **What fungus produces a granulomatous tissue reaction and can cause the triad of pneumonitis, erythema nodosum and arthralgias known as valley fever?**

Coccidioidomycosis.

O   **Up to 50% of pulmonary arteriovenous malformations are associated with what inherited disorder?**

Hereditary hemorrhagic telangiectasia (Osler-Weber-Rendu Disease).

O   *A chest xray of a smoker reveals a popcorn lesion. This slow growing tumor is needle biopsied (sensitiv) and the diagnosis is?*

Hamartoma.

O   **At what rate will the intrapleural air of a pneumothorax be reabsorbed if left untreated?**

1.25% per day.

○   **What are the disadvantages associated with treating a pneumothorax with catheter aspiration alone?**

It is difficult to evacuate the entire pneumothorax and it is not applicable in patients with an active air leak.

○   **Through what interspace should a chest tube be inserted for treatment of a pneumothorax?**

The fourth or fifth intercostal space.

○   **What complications are seen from chest tubes placed too low on the chest wall?**

Injury to the diaphragm or abdominal viscera.

○   **What is the most common type of pleural effusion in infants?**

Chylothorax.

○   **What are the indications for surgical treatment of a chylothorax?**

Failure of nonoperative therapy after 7 to 14 days, continued drainage of more that 1,500 ml/day in adults, persistent electrolyte abnormalities and/or malnutrition.

○   **T/F: Ligation of the thoracic duct at the diaphragmatic hiatus can be performed without significant side effects.**

True.

○   **If during the operative treatment of a chylothorax, the site of leakage cannot be identified, what definitive procedure should be performed?**

Ligation of the thoracic duct at the diaphragm.

○   **What is the most common location of the thoracic duct at the level of the diaphragm?**

Between the aorta and the vertebral bodies.

○   **What volume of pleural fluid is needed to obliterate the costophrenic angle on chest x-ray?**

250 ml.

○   *A man receives a stab to his lower neck/ chest. At the junction of L IJ and subclavian. A chest tube is placed revealing milky white fluid. What is the treatment of this injury?*

Chest tube drainage and npo x 2 wks. If this does not resolve then thoracotomy and thoracic duct ligation.

○   **Where does the thoracic duct enter the chest?**

Enters on right at T12 and traverses to the right of the aorta. It crosses the midline to join at IJ/Sucblavian junction

○   **What is the most common metastatic tumor to produce a malignant pleural effusion?**

Breast cancer.

○   **What is the initial management of refractory malignant pleural effusions not relieved by chemotherapy or radiation of the primary tumor?**

Thoracostomy tube drainage followed by talc or chemical pleurodesis.

❍   **T/F: Most pleuroperitoneal shunts occlude soon after placement, precluding successful palliation in patients with malignant pleural effusions.**

False.

❍   **What percentage of patients with middle lobe syndrome have bronchiectasis?**

40%.

❍   **What type of pulmonary resection is most frequently associated with postoperative empyema?**

Pneumonectomy (2 to 12%).

❍   **What percentage of patients requiring extracorporeal membrane oxygenation (ECMO) develop an intracranial bleed?**

66%.

❍   *A tall thin male presents with SOB. A CXR reveals a Pneumothorax. What are the chances it will recur? And what should be done on recurrence?*

Spontaneous pneumothorax - 50% recur and of those that recur. Thoracoscopy with pleurodesis for recurrence or continuous air leak.

❍   *When should patients with myasthenia gravis (MG) undergo thymectomy?*

As soon as possible after the development of generalized weakness.

❍   *When is lung decortication indicated in the treatment of empyema?*

When a residual undrained space prevents complete lung re-expansion, in spite of less invasive measures (i.e., tube thoracostomy with or without fibrinolytic enzymes or thoracoscopic debridement).

❍   **What is an Eloesser flap procedure?**

An open drainage procedure for an empyema cavity.

❍   **What options remain for a persistent empyema cavity that cannot be sterilized by open drainage or irrigation?**

Decortication, obliteration of the pleural space using muscle flaps or omentum, thoracoplasty or the Claggett procedure.

❍   **T/F: Pleural pneumonectomy for malignant mesothelioma has been shown to increase overall patient survival when compared to chemotherapy or radiation therapy.**

False.

❍   **What conditions are consistently associated with pectus excavatum?**

Marfan's syndrome, mitral valve prolapse and scoliosis.

❍   **What pulmonary function parameters are significantly improved following pectus excavatum repair?**

Total lung capacity (TLC) and maximal voluntary ventilation. (MVV).

○ **T/F: Following chest wall resection, skeletal defects located near the tip of the scapula should always be reconstructed.**

True.

○ **What are the preferred materials for reconstructing skeletal defects following chest wall resection?**

2 mm-thick polytetrafluorethylene or a customized solid plate made of polypropylene mesh and methylmethacrylate.

○ **When should decortication be considered in treating a hemothorax that is refractory to chest tube drainage?**

When a significant collection persists in spite of tube thoracosotomy, intrapleural fibrinolytic enzymes and thoracoscopic debridement.

○ **When postoperative infection is excluded, what etiology is responsible for approximately 90% of cases of acute mediastinitis?**

Esophageal perforation.

○ **What is the treatment for descending necrotizing mediastinitis?**

Broad spectrum antibiotics and wide surgical drainage, usually requiring neck and transthoracic drainage, with frequent reevaluation for possible undrained collections.

○ **Why is it important to obtain a tissue diagnosis prior to treating superior vena cava syndrome in all patients?**

High dose radiation therapy may alter the tumor's histology and prevent a subsequent accurate diagnosis. It is also important to identify benign conditions and tumors that may respond to chemotherapy or radiation therapy.

○ *A thin man with lung cancer presents with facial swelling and jvd and sob. What is the treatment?*

SVC syndrome - most commonly caused by lung cancer. It is treated initially by radiation therapy.

○ **Masses located in the middle or posterior mediastinum are best resected through what type of incision?**

A posterolateral thoracotomy.

○ **What surgical technique is useful for evaluation and biopsy of a mass of the middle mediastinum?**

Mediastinoscopy.

○ **What special anesthetic considerations are necessary before induction of patients with large anterior or middle mediastinal masses?**

Airway compression and vascular collapse.

○ **How should neurogenic mediastinal tumors involving the spinal cord be resected?**

One stage resection of the intraspinal and thoracic components.

○ **What percentage of patients with MG are found to have a thymoma on chest CT or MRI?**

10 to 42%.

○   **What is the treatment of choice for patients with a thymoma?**

Complete surgical excision of the thymus with postoperative radiation therapy for invasive tumors (stage II or III).

○   **Modern differentiation between benign and malignant thymic tumors is based on what factors?**

Presence of gross invasion of adjacent structures at the time of surgery, presence of metastases and microscopic evidence of capsular invasion.

○   **T/F: Anterosuperior mediastinal masses in adults are most often malignant.**

True.

○   **T/F: Enteric mediastinal cysts are not routinely excised.**

False.

LIVER, GALLBLADDER, PANCREAS AND SPLEEN PEARLS

Confirmed dispepsia is the apparatus of illusions.
George Meredith

O   **What is the mechanism of hypotension in severe cases of acute pancreatitis?**

Fluid sequestration in the intestine and retroperitoneum, systemic vascular effects of kinins, vomiting and bleeding.

O   **What is the pathological spectrum of acute pancreatitis?**

Edematous pancreatitis to necrotizing pancreatitis.

O   **T/F: Idiopathic acute pancreatitis may be the result of occult biliary microlithiasis or biliary sludge.**

True.

O   **What is the most common type of lipid profile seen in pancreatitis?**

Type V (increased triglycerides).

O   **How does excess lipid promote pancreatitis?**

By the toxic action of fatty acids released by lipase in the pancreas.

O   **What is the mechanism of necrosis and vascular damage in acute pancreatitis?**

Autodigestion of the pancreas by various proteolytic and lipolytic enzymes.

O   **What is the role of abdominal ultrasound in pancreatitis?**

Detection of biliary obstruction and regression of pseudocysts.

O   **What are the criteria for severity in nonbiliary pancreatitis at 48 hours?**

Fall in hematocrit greater than 10%, rise in BUN greater than 5% per mg/dl, serum calcium less than 8 mg/dl, PaO2 less than 60 mm Hg, base deficit greater than 4 mEq/l and fluid sequestration greater than 6 liters.

O   **What are the criteria for severity in biliary pancreatitis on admission?**

Age greater than 70 years, WBC greater than 18/mm3, glucose greater than 220 mg/dl, LDH greater than 400 U/l and AST greater than 250 U/l.

O   ***Should antibiotics be given emperically to patients with severe pancreatitis?***

Yes.

O   **What are the signs and symptoms of the complications of pancreatitis?**

Persistent fever, leukocytosis, pain, tenderness and overall clinical deterioration.

O   **What is the mortality of acute pancreatitis?**

1% for those with 2 or less factors by the Ranson's criteria, 16% for 3 or 4, 40% for 5 or 6 and 100% for those with 7 or 8 factors.

O   *What are the most common variants in origin of hepatic arteries?*

Right hepatic- Off SMA-20%.
Left hepatic- Off Left Gastic-10%.

O   **What are the structures in portal triad?**

Portal vein- most posterior.
CBD- on the right.
Hepatic artery- on the left.

O   **T/F: The portal vein formed by the SMV and splenic VV sees highly regulated blood flow with its multiple valves.**

False. The portal system is valveless.

O   **What pleuropulmonary abnormalities may be seen in patients with pancreatitis?**

Elevated hemidiaphragm, atelectasis, pleural reaction or effusion, hypoxemia and acute lung injury, including ARDS.

O   **When should surgical drainage of pancreatic pseudocysts be considered?**

In patients with large cysts (greater than 5 cm) and those with cysts that do not resolving or decrease within 6 weeks of onset.

O   **What is the appropriate treatment for patients with chronic pancreatitis?**

Supportive.

O   **After Cholecytectomy pathology reveals an adenocarcinoma. The Ca is confined to the mucosa (T1). What are the options?**

Cholecytectomy is sufficient.

O   *What is the treatment for a T3 adenocarcinoma of the gallbladder?*

Cholecystectomy + Regional lymphadenectomy and liver segment V removal, and portal triad Skeletonization.

O   **An arteriogram is done to work up hematobilia. Hematobilia consists of which triad?**

GI bleed, Jaundice, RUQ pain.

O   **What factors affect liver blood flow during anesthesia?**

Hypoxemia, hypercarbia, hypovolemia and sympathetic stimulation. Surgical retraction of the liver can be a major factor in decreasing liver blood flow.

O   **What are the effects of CO_2 on liver blood flow?**

Hypocarbia decreases hepatic arterial blood flow. Hypercarbia increases portal and total hepatic arterial blood flow.

O **What is the role of the liver during acute hemorrhage?**

The liver may act as a reservoir of blood (up to 500 ml).

O *What does charcot's triad imply.*

Fever, RUQ tenderness and jaundice is indicative of Cholangitis.
Adding hypotension and mental status changes= renolds pentad.
Tx: Iv abx, IVF, and emergent drainage of biliary tract.

O **What is the most common cause of biliary stricture?**

Iatrogenic injury (lap chole).

O **What are the dangers of porcelin Gallbladder?**

Risk of cancer is 30-65%. Therefore mandatory cholecystecyomy.

O **Pt complains of RUQ pain yet has no gall stones. CCK stimulation reveals a EF < 35% what is the diagnosis?**

Biliary dyskinesia and hence indication for cholycystectomy.

O **What is the rule of 10's for insulinomas?**

10% solitary.
10% malignant.
10% associated with MEN.
10% ectopic.

O **What are the typical hemodynamic changes seen in cirrhosis?**

A hyperdynamic circulation with an increase in cardiac output (CO) and a decrease in systemic vascular resistance (SVR).

O **Why is CO increased in patients with liver disease?**

Peripheral vasodilatation and arteriovenous shunting.

O **What is the effect of cirrhosis on mixed venous oxygen saturation?**

It is increased.

O *What is the most common site of obstruction in gallstone ileus?*

The terminal ileum.

O **What are the causes of hypoxia in patients with chronic liver disease?**

Ventilation/perfusion (V/Q) mismatching, intrapulmonary and portopulmonary shunting, limitation of alveolar-capillary diffusion, loss of hypoxic vasoconstriction and a rightward shift of the oxyhemoglobin dissociation curve.

O **What is the association between portal hypertension and pulmonary hypertension?**

There is a small (less than 2%) but definite association.

O   **Is the blood volume increased or decreased in cirrhosis?**
This is highly controversial. There is certainly an altered distribution of fluids with a decrease in circulating or effective blood volume.

O   **T/F: Amebic abscess of liver a treated with Metronidazole?**

True.

O   **What is the normal pancreatic anatomy and in pts with pancreas divisum?**

NL- Santorini= small   Wirsung= Major.
Divisum Santorini= Major duct.
Divisum occurs in 5% pop and is failure of embryologic failure of fusion of ducts. These patients are prone to pancreatitis.

O   **What gene is mutated in 90% of pancreatic cancer pts?**

K-Ras.

O   **What is the Most common islet cell tumor?**

Insulinoma.

O   *What is the surgical of insulinoma?*

Enucleation.

O   **What is the appropriate management of the hepatorenal syndrome (HRS)?**

Recognition and correction of prerenal factors often improves the overall renal function.

O   *What are Antithrombin III, protein C and protein S? What is their importance in patients with liver disease?*

These are inhibitors of coagulation, deficiency of which may lead to thrombotic states. They are synthesized in the liver and may be decreased in patients with cirrhosis. However, these patients do not usually have a thrombotic state due to a concomitant decrease in coagulation factors.

O   **T/F: Regional anesthesia is contraindicated in patients with a coagulopathy.**

True.

O   **What are the immediate hemodynamic effects upon release of a portocaval shunt?**

An increase in right atrial and pulmonary capillary pressures and a decrease in SVR.

O   *Why do cirrhotic patients develop prolonged apnea after succinylcholine administration?*

They have a decreased synthesis of pseudocholinesterase.

O   **Which shunts are appropriate for the treatment of patients with Budd-Chiari syndrome?**

Side-to-side portocaval, mesocaval and mesoatrial.

❍   *A 45 year old cirrhotic patient undergoing portocaval shunt has profuse surgical bleeding. Transfusion of red blood cells (RBCs) and fresh frozen plasma (FFP) is in progress. The patient is hypotensive in spite of adequate replacement of intravascular volume. What is the most likely cause?*

Hypocalcemia.

❍   **How is coagulopathy managed in patients scheduled for surgery?**

Administration of vitamin K and cryoprecipitate, infusion of FFP for an INR less than 1.5 and transfusion of platelets to levels above 100,000/mm³.

❍   **What is the most appropriate treatment for a patient with choledocholithiasis 2 years after cholecystectomy?**

Endoscopic sphincterotomy and stone extraction.

❍   **What are the cardiovascular implications of alcoholic liver disease during anesthesia?**

Overt or subclinical cadiomyopathy and decreased responsiveness to epinephrine.

❍   **T/F: Intracranial pressure (ICP) is increased in patients with fulminant hepatic failure (FHF).**

True.

❍   **What drugs are effective if spasm of the sphincter of Oddi is suspected?**

Atropine, glucagon, naloxone and nitroglycerin.

❍   **What are important anesthetic considerations specific to OLT?**

Hemodynamic perturbation and a potential for major blood loss in patients with preexisting coagulopathy.

❍   **How is venovenous bypass different from cardiopulmonary bypass?**

During venovenous bypass, blood from the lower part of the body and the portal circulation is returned to the axillary or jugular veins via a centrifugal pump. An oxygenator is generally not used and heparinization is not required during venovenous bypass.

❍   **What type of gallstone is associated with cirrhosis and hemolysis?**

Black-pigment stones (bilirubin).

❍   *Where is an accessory right hepatic artery found and what is its origin?*

It can arise from the superior mesenteric artery and passes posterior to the head of the pancreas, to the right of the portal vein and posterior to the common bile duct (seen in 15-20% of patients).

❍   **When is it not safe to ligate the gastroduodenal artery?**

When the gastroduodenal artery is the hepatic artery and arises from the superior mesenteric artery.

❍   **Which bifurcation occurs first in the hilum of the liver: hepatic artery, portal vein or common hepatic duct?**

The hepatic artery.

❍   **Is preservation of the hepatic veins important in hepatic resection?**

Usually not. There are connections between the hepatic veins, as long as one of them is left open, the venous drainage of the remnant is generally adequate.

O   **How is the diagnosis of amebic abscess confirmed?**

By indirect hemagglutination.

O   **What pathologic features of hepatocellular carcinoma (HCC) are associated with improved survival?**

Tumors exhibiting the fibrolamellar variant, encapsulated tumors and pedunculated tumors.

O   **What is total vascular exclusion as used for liver resection?**

Control and occlusion of the hepatic artery, portal vein and supra- and infrahepatic vena cava to allow hepatic parenchymal transection in a bloodless field.

O   **What is partial vascular exclusion as used for liver resection?**

Control and occlusion of the inflow and outflow to the resected portions of the liver during hepatic parenchymal transection to reduce blood loss.

O   **What is intermittent ischemia as applied to liver resection?**

The inflow of the liver is periodically occluded for brief periods of time (typically 15 to 20 minutes). The liver is then reperfused for 5 minutes before the clamp is reapplied. Total occlusion times of up to 200 minutes have been reported without mortality.

O   **What factors increase the likelihood of curative liver resection for metastatic colorectal cancer to the liver?**

Long interval between resection of the primary and discovery of the liver metastasis and ability to resect lesion(s) with a l cm margin of normal tissue.

O   **What is the cure rate for resectable liver metastases from a colon primary?**

20 to 30%.

O   **T/F: Hepatic artery infusion of chemotherapy increases survival in patients with hepatic metastases from colon and rectal primaries.**

False.

O   *What is the appropriate treatment for a patient with a 6 cm calcified cystic lesion in the anterior right lobe of the liver with a positive Casoni test?*

Pericystectomy.

O   **What techniques are available to limit the number of patients subjected to operation who ultimately prove to have incurable and/or unresectable liver metastases?**

CT angiography, MRI, PET scan, laparoscopic ultrasound and exploration.

O   **T/F: Cryoablation is an alternative to curative liver resection for hepatic metastases.**

False. Cryosurgery is currently only a palliative treatment.

O   *What drug is associated with hepatic adenomas and what is there treatment?*

Estrogen, surgical resection is Tx.

O   *How often does cancer arise in focal nodular hyperplasia?*

Virtually never.

O   **What is the 5-year survival rate following resection of hepatocellular carcinoma in a noncirrhotic liver?**

30%.

O   **What are the indications for surgery for patients with cavernous hemangioma of the liver?**

Pain due to hemorrhage or rupture and development of a consumptive coagulopathy.

O   **If a hepatic cyst compresses the biliary tree or contains bile, how is the treatment of the cyst different?**

Sclerosis of the cyst should not be undertaken if there is evidence of involvement of the biliary tree as secondary sclerosing cholangitis may result.

O   **T/F: Cytology of hepatic cyst contents reliably predicts the presence or absence of tumor in the cyst lining.**

False.

O   **What is the most common cause of death from adult polycystic liver disease?**

Cerebrovascular accident from an aneurysm or complications of renal failure.

O   **What is the treatment of choice for hydatid cysts of the liver?**

Radical removal of the cyst including the pericyst (sclerotic, fibrous reactive capsule).

O   **What are the immediate risks of peritoneovenous shunting?**

A disseminated thrombolytic state may result from infusion of ascitic fluid. If renal function is insufficient, CHF may result from the infusion of a large volume of peritoneal fluid. In addition, infected peritoneal fluid will result in sepsis if a shunt is placed before adequate treatment is completed.

O   **T/F: Malignant ascites is a contraindication of peritoneovenous shunting.**

False.

O   **What is the Sigura procedure?**

An operation for bleeding esophageal varices in which division of the esophageal varices is accomplished by transection of the esophagus and reanastomosis, usually with an EEA stapler.

O   **In what way does extrahepatic portal hypertension differ from portal hypertension in the most common setting of post necrotic cirrhosis?**

Usually, extrahepatic portal hypertension is the result of thrombosis of the portal or splenic vein.

O   *What is the proper treatment for bleeding gastric varices without esophageal varices?*

Splenectomy for splenic vein thrombosis.

○   **What are the key issues in management of patients with portal hypertension resulting from Budd-Chiari syndrome?**

Patency of the IVC and quality of liver function.

○   **When is surgical shunting indicted?**

For patients with extrahepatic portal hypertension or with well-compensated cirrhosis (Child's class A).

○   **What is the most common cause of portal hypertension in children?**

Portal vein thrombosis.

○   **What pressure defines portal hypertension and why?**

12 mm Hg is generally accepted as portal hypertension. Below this level, bleeding from varices is rarely seen.

○   **What substances are thought to be responsible for the hyperdynamic circulation seen in patients with cirrhosis and portal hypertension?**

Prostaglandins, glucagon, nitric oxide and tumor necrosis factor (TNF).

○   **What is the role of transjugular intrahepatic portosystemic shunting (TIPS) in the management of variceal hemorrhage?**

TIPS is a temporary shunt that functions as a small diameter end-to-side shunt. The expected duration of the shunt is 6 months to 2 years. It is most suited to management of variceal hemorrhage in patients not responding to banding or sclerotherapy and those with gastric varices. It is an excellent bridge to transplantation for those who might not tolerate a surgical shunt and who are candidates for liver transplantation.

○   **What are the therapeutic approaches to hepatic encephalopathy?**

Oral antibiotics and lactulose.

○   **What is the importance of the Child's classification?**

It stratifies patients with liver disease according to the severity of derangement of the following factors: encephalopathy, nutrition, ascites, bilirubin, albumin and prothrombin time. The severity of the Child's classification predicts surgical outcome.

○   **What are the characteristic features of beta-thalassemia major?**

Persistence of Hb-F and a reduction in Hb-A.

○   **What are the characteristic laboratory findings in a patient with idiopathic thrombocytopenia purpura (ITP)?**

A platelet count of less than 50,000/mm3, prolonged bleeding time and a normal clotting time.

○   *What is the treatment for ITP?*

An initial 6 weeks to 2 month's trial of steroids. If there is no response to steroid therapy, splenectomy is indicated.

○   **What is the mechanism of portal hypertension caused by schistosomiasis?**

Presinusoidal obstruction.

○   **A 30 year old female presents with acute onset of fever and purpura. Laboratory evaluation reveals anemia, thrombocytopenia, leukocytosis and an elevated BUN and creatinine. What is the most likely diagnosis?**

Thrombotic thrombocytopenic purpura (TTP).

○   **What enzyme level is most likely to be decreased in a 50 kg woman with cholesterol gallstones?**
7-alpha-hydroxylase.

○   **When is splenectomy indicated in patients with myeloid metaplasia?**

For control of anemia and thrombocytopenia and for symptoms of splenomegaly.

○   **What are the characteristic blood smear findings of a post-splenectomy patient?**

Howell-Jolly bodies, siderocytes, leukocytosis and an increased platelet count.

○   **What are the most common causes of spontaneous splenic rupture?**

Complications of malaria and mononucleosis.

○   **What is the appropriate management for patients with portal vein injury that cannot be repaired?**

Ligation of the portal vein.

○   **What is the pathophysiology of TTP?**

Occlusion of capillaries and arterioles.

○   **What are the most common causes of secondary hypersplenism?**

Hepatic disease or extrahepatic portal vein obstruction.

○   **T/F: Splenectomy is the treatment of choice for patients with hairy cell leukemia.**

False. Splenectomy is reserved for patients who fail medical management.

○   **What class of splenic injury exists when there is an expanding subcapsular hematoma?**

Class III.

○   **What is the inheritance pattern of hereditary spherocytosis?**

Autosomal dominant.

○   **What percentage of the pancreatic blood flow goes to the islets of Langerhans?**

20%.

○   *What are the clinical manifestations of pancreatic exocrine insufficiency?*

Steatorrhea and malabsorption.

○   **What is the typical clinical course of sclerosing cholangitis?**

Chronic, relapsing disease associated with jaundice, pruritis, pain and fatigue.

O   **What percentages of alcoholics develop chronic pancreatitis?**

10 to 15%.

O   **What is the significance of Gray Turner's syndrome?**

This represents dissection of blood from the retroperitoneum near the pancreas in patients with hemorrhagic pancreatitis.

O   **What would you expect the serum amylase level to be in a patient with acute pancreatitis?**

2 to 5 times normal.

O   **What veins are ligated during a distal splenorenal shunt?**

The inferior mesenteric vein, coronary vein and pancreatic branches of the splenic vein.

O   **What is the most common finding on plain abdominal x-ray in a patient with acute pancreatitis?**

Dilatation of an isolated loop of intestine adjacent to the pancreas (sentinel loop).

O   **A 60 year old male presents to the emergency room with acute pancreatitis. His WBC count is 14,000/mm3, blood glucose is 250 mg/dl, LDH is 400 and his AST is 275. What is his mortality risk?**

15% (3 ranson's criteria present).

O   **What is the most common cause of death in patients with adenocarcinoma of the extrahepatic bile ducts?**

Hepatic failure and sepsis from biliary obstruction.

O   **What is the principle symptom in the majority of patients with chronic pancreatitis?**

Abdominal pain, usually in the epigastrum and described as cramping, boring or aching.

O   **What are the most common complications of chronic pancreatitis?**

Pseudocyst, diabetes mellitus (DM) and malnutrition.

O   **Pt has severe ulcer, diarrhea, and gastrin > 1000. In addition secretin stimulation test results in elevated gastrin level. What is your diagnosis?**

Gastrinoma.

O   **What is the Most common islet cell tumor in MEN I?**

Gastrinoma.

O   **Where are 90% gastrinomas located?**

Gastrinoma triangle.- cystic/ cbd junction-pancreas neck-3rd portion duodenum.

O   ***What medical conditions are associated with somatostatinoma?***

Gallstones, steatorrhea, pancreatitis, diabetes.

❍ *What skin condition is associated with Glucogonoma?*

Migratory necrolytic erythema.

❍ *What syndrome is associated with VIP oma?*

WHADA syndrome= watery diarrhea hypokalemia achlorhydria.

❍ *T/F: NGT and H2 blockers improve symptoms in Gastrinoma and VIP oma?*

False. Will improve gastrinoma symptoms only.

❍ **When should a lateral pancreaticojejunostomy (Puestow procedure) be performed?**

When the diameter of the main pancreatic duct increases to 7 mm or more.

❍ **When should pancreatic resection be considered?**

For patients with severe pain, when the pancreatic duct is narrow or normal, patients who have recurrence following the Puestow procedure and for patients with pathologic changes in the pancreas.

❍ **What are the absolute indications for common bile duct exploration at the time of cholecystectomy?**

Palpable or cholangiographic evidence of a stone in the duct and the presence of cholangitis.

❍ **What is the appropriate medical treatment for a patient with acute hemorrhage from esophageal varices, following resuscitation?**

Intravenous vasopressin.

❍ **What is the best method to assess the risk of bleeding from esophageal varices?**

The size of the varices when viewed endoscopically.

❍ **What type of cancer accounts for 90% of exocrine pancreatic tumors?**

Ductal adenocarcinoma.

❍ **What is the mortality rate for patients with pancreatic ductal adenocarcinoma?**

Greater than 95%.

❍ **What is meant by a modified Whipple?**

Preservation of the stomach and pylorus.

❍ **What is the most common benign neoplasm of the exocrine pancreas?**

Serous (microcystic) cystadenomas.

❍ **What is the best test for confirmation of the diagnosis of insulinoma?**

Demonstration of fasting hypoglycemia in the face of an inappropriately high level of insulin.

❍ **What percentage of gastrinomas are solitary adenomas?**

25%.

❍   **What are the laboratory requirements for the diagnosis of gastrinoma?**

Fasting hypergastrinemia (greater than 200 pg/ml blood) in the face of gastric acid hypersecretion (basal acid output greater than 15 mEq/hr) with an intact stomach or greater than 5 mEq/hr after ulcer surgery.

❍   *If a patient has a serum gastrin level of 200 to 500 pg/ml, what test must be done to confirm the diagnosis of gastrinoma?*

The secretin provocative test.

❍   *What is the drug of choice for the treatment of gastrinoma?*

Omeprazole.

❍   *What is the cause of most cases of WDHA (Watery Diarrhea, Hypokalemia and Achlorhydria)?*

An islet cell tumor of the pancreas that produces vasoactive intestinal polypeptide (VIP).

❍   *What conditions are associated with annular pancreas?*

Down's syndrome, duodenal atresia and peptic ulcer.

❍   *A 53 year old alcoholic patient presents to the emergency room with pancreatitis and 5 of Ranson's criteria. What is the initial treatment of this patient?*

Gastric decompression and intravenous antibiotics. APO status and TPN as well.

❍   **What is the most appropriate treatment for a patient who presents with acute gallstone pancreatitis?**

Initial ERCP with papillotomy, subsequent cholecystectomy.

❍   **What are the biochemical characteristics of pancreatic ascites?**

Fluid amylase greater than serum amylase and fluid protein greater than 2.5 gm/dl.

❍   *What is the most appropriate treatment for a 55 year old alcoholic with chronic pancreatitis, intractable abdominal pain and no evidence of diabetes?*

Lateral pancreaticojejunostomy if the pancreatic duct is dilated.

❍   **What is the function of ceruloplasmin?**

It binds and transports copper.

❍   **What is the most common type of biliary enteric fistula?**

Cholecystoduodenal.

❍   **Which benign hepatic lesions are associated with exogenous estrogen use?**

Hemangiomas, hepatic adenomas and focal nodular hyperplasia (FNH).

❍   **A 27 year old female undergoes exploration for a benign appearing large, solitary hepatic cyst after experiencing progressive RUQ pain. Upon unroofing the cyst, frozen section of the cyst wall reveals a cuboidal epithelial lining. Is any further treatment indicated?**

Yes. A wedge resection or lobectomy should be performed for definitive resection.

❍   **What is the most common manifestation of decompensation in a cirrhotic patient?**

Ascites.

❍   **What is the mortality rate for an initial variceal hemorrhage?**

40 to 50%.

❍   **What are the characteristics of Type I FHF?**

Hepatocellular necrosis and markedly elevated transaminases.

❍   **How does prerenal azotemia result from the medical management of cirrhosis?**

Diuretics used for ascites and peripheral edema can contract intravascular volume, resulting in prerenal azotemia.

❍   **What benign hepatic lesion is characterized by the presence of Kupffer cells?**

Focal nodular hyperplasia.

❍   **What gallbladder tumor is neuroectodermally derived?**

Granular cell myoblastoma.

❍   **What is the most common benign hepatic tumor?**

Cavernous hemangiomas.

❍   **What clinical finding is characteristic of hepatocellular carcinoma?**

Painful hepatomegaly.

❍   **During laparoscopic cholecystectomy for a 32 year old female, multiple thin adhesions are seen in the right upper quadrant to the surface of the liver and surrounding the fundus of the gallbladder. What is the presumed etiology?**

Fitz Hugh-Curtis syndrome.

❍   **T/F: There is an association between the presence of gallstones and the occurrence of gallbladder adenocarcinoma.**

True. 70% of cases of gallbladder adenocarcinoma occur in patients with long-standing cholelithiasis.

❍   **What is the name for a cholangiocarcinoma that presents at the confluence of the right and left hepatic ducts?**

A Klatskin tumor.

❍   **ERCP performed for a non-alcoholic patient with recurrent pancreatitis reveals that the predominant drainage of the pancreas is via the lesser duct. What is the most likely diagnosis?**

Pancreas divisum.

❍   **T/F: A patient with a mass in the tail of the pancreas undergoes distal pancreatectomy with resection of 60% of the gland. Postoperative complications include diabetes.**

False.

❍   **What is the common channel concept in relation to obstructive pancreatitis?**

A portion of the common bile duct is shared with the main pancreatic duct in 66% of the population. Passage of gallstones may obstruct at this level, leading to the development of acute pancreatitis with biliary reflux into the pancreatic duct, which is thought to be a contributing factor.

❍   **What percentage of patients develop severe pancreatitis following routine ERCP.**

1%.

❍   **A 60 year old male presents with severe abdominal pain. He as a WBC count of 18,000/mm3 and a serum glucose 250 mg/dl on admission. Within 24 hours his hematocrit has dropped 10% and his serum calcium is 6 mg/dl. What is his estimated mortality from acute pancreatitis?**

40% (4 ranson's crieteria).

❍   *What is the pathognomonic finding for chronic pancreatitis on KUB?*

Pancreatic calcifications.

❍   *A 47 year old male presents with an epigastric mass, early satiety and weight loss. His history is significant for an episode of alcohol-induced pancreatitis six months ago and his serum amylase is normal. What is the most likely diagnosis and what is the optimal treatment ?*

A pancreatic pseudocyst. Treatment is enteric drainage if unresolving or causing significant symptoms.

❍   **What are the indications for surgical intervention for a patient with a pancreatic pseudocyst?**

Size greater than 5 cm, infection, gastrointestinal obstruction, hemorrhage, spontaneous rupture and failure to resolve within 6 weeks, given adequate conservative management.

❍   **A 57 year old male with long standing chronic pancreatitis gradually experiences relief of pain without medical intervention. What is the most likely diagnosis?**

Progressive fibrosis of the gland with complete pancreatic exocrine insufficiency.

❍   **A 68 year old male presents with vague, recurrent abdominal pain. What is the most sensitive and specific test for the diagnosis of chronic pancreatitis?**

ERCP.

❍   **What are the surgical indications for chronic pancreatitis?**

Intractable pain with lifestyle changes, inability to work and narcotic addiction.

❍   **What are the indications for pancreatic resection versus pancreatic drainage?**

Drainage is an option if the pancreatic ducts are dilated beyond 8 mm. Resection is indicated if the ducts are small or if they are of normal caliber when an isolated portion of the gland is affected. Resection is also indicated after a failed drainage procedure.

O   **A patient has failed to get adequate pain relief from a Peustow procedure. What is the next procedure of choice?**

Pancreaticoduodenectomy. Consider celiac nerve block if multiple co-morbidities.

O   **What are the relative contraindications to peritoneovenous shunting for intractable ascites?**

Acute hepatitis, uncorrectable coagulopathy and history of variceal bleeding.

O   **A 50 year old female, who consumes ETOH occasionally, presents with a stricture of the CBD that appears as an abrupt termination of contrast on ERCP. What is the most likely diagnosis?**

Malignancy.

O   **A 37 year old male, with known chronic pancreatitis, presents with isolated elevation of alkaline phosphatase. What are the indications for operative repair of a biliary stricture related to chronic pancreatitis?**

Cholangitis, cirrhotic changes on liver biopsy, persistent jaundice, inability to rule out malignancy, progression of the stricture and persistent elevation of alkaline phosphatase greater than 3 times normal.

O   **A patient develops a pancreatic fistula 13 days following pancreaticoduodenectomy. What is the appropriate treatment?**

Re-operation.

O   **A 58 year old male develops a moderate amount of bleeding from a drain site 24 hours after a Whipple resection. What catastrophic complication does this represent?**

A necrotizing retroperitoneal infection with erosion into an exposed portal vein.

O   **In choosing a partial versus complete pancreatectomy, what is the rationale for total pancreatectomy for patients with an exocrine neoplasms of the pancreas?**

The eradication of residual disease at margins of resection and avoidance of pancreaticojejunostomy with risk of disruption.

O   **In what situations should the gallbladder be utilized, rather than the common bile duct, in the creation of a biliary bypass for palliation in unresectable pancreatic carcinoma?**

Invasion of the porta hepatis by tumor, presence of a bulky tumor precluding use of the common bile duct, poor patient status and portal vein thrombosis with periductal varices.

O   **During a palliative procedure for unresectable pancreatic carcinoma, aspiration of the gallbladder returns clear fluid. What does this indicate?**

Complete cystic duct occlusion.

O   **A 33 year old female presents with vague abdominal discomfort and a palpable abdominal mass. Imaging studies reveal a 10 cm mass in the tail of the pancreas with solid and cystic components. What is the most likely diagnosis and treatment?**

This is likely a tumor and is treated with distal pancreatectomy with a 90% cure rate.

O   **What would the same scenario indicate in a 70 year old female?**

A serous cystadenoma or cystadenocarcinoma. Treatment would also be resection.

❍   **What are the contraindications to performing a portocaval shunt?**

Portal vein thrombosis and a large caudate lobe of the liver.

❍   *Which pancreatic exocrine neoplasm most closely resembles a pancreatic pseudocyst?*

Mucinous cystadenoma.

❍   **What is the best method to find an elusive insulinoma when there is preoperative laboratory based confirmation of its presence?**

Endoscopic ultrasound.

❍   **What endoscopic finding is the hallmark of Zollinger-Ellsion syndrome?**

Peptic ulcerations in an unusual site, including postbulbar and jejunal ulcerations.

❍   *If a patient presents with severe refractory PUD and diarrhea, what test should be done to rule out gastrinoma?*

The secretin stimulation test.

❍   **What is the initial treatment for patients with pancreatitis?**

NPO until near complete resolution of pain and tenderness.

❍   *What is the appropriate treatment of a type I choledochal cyst?*

Cyst excision with roux-en-y hepatico-jejunostomy.

❍   **What are the indications for gallstone dissolution therapy?**

Stones that are less than 5 mm and noncalcified and a gallbladder that opacifies on oral cholecystogram (indicating patency of the cystic duct). Dissolution therapy, commonly with ursodiol, is effective in dissolving 50% of stones within 2 years.

❍   **What vein enters the retrohepatic vena cava (other than the hepatic veins)?**

The right adrenal vein.

❍   **Where are primary bile salts converted to secondary bile salts?**

In the small intestine.

❍   **What are the complications of total portosystemic shunts?**

Encephalopathy and hepatic failure.

❍   **What is the significance of delta bilirubin?**

It accumulates in large quantities in patients with chronic conjugated hyperbilirubinemia and persists after the underlying problem is corrected and the bound albumin is metabolized.

❍   **How is the endothelial lining of the hepatic sinusoid different from other capillaries and what is its significance?**

It has large fenestrations. Consequently, it has a permeability of about 30 times that of other capillaries. Thus, filtration through the sinusoid is much faster. In addition, there is a space on the tissue side of the sinusoid (the space of Disse) giving the hepatocyte a large surface for contact with the filtered fluid in the extravascular space.

○   **What are the elements of Charcot's triad?**

Jaundice, fever with chills and biliary colic.

○   **What organisms are most commonly involved in bacterial cholangitis?**

E. coli, klebsiella, pseudomonas, enterococci and proteus.

○   **What are the common complications of choledocholithiasis?**

Secondary biliary cirrhosis, acute pancreatitis and intrahepatic abscesses.

○   **How is the caudate lobe different from the other segments of the liver, with respect to its vascular supply?**

It receives blood from the right and left hepatic arteries and the portal vein. Most of the venous blood drains directly into the vena cava.

○   **What percentage of normal persons have classic hepatic arterial anatomy (a single hepatic artery arising from the celiac axis and dividing into the left and right hepatic arteries)?**

50%.

○   *What therapy is indicated for an amebic abscess?*

Metronidazole, 400 mg TID for 4 days or a single dose of 2.5 gm, combined with aspiration.

○   **What are the risk factors for hepatocellular carcinoma (HCC)?**

Aflatoxins, low protein intake, hepatitis B and C and cirrhosis.

○   **How is alpha-fetoprotein (AFP) helpful in following patients with cirrhosis for the development of cancer?**

A rising AFP predicts development of HCC.

○   **How does cirrhosis affect the outcome of liver resection?**

The cirrhotic liver regenerates poorly and may not fully recover after extensive liver resection. Hepatic failure may ensue.

○   **What intraoperative factors can influence the outcome of liver resection in the cirrhotic patient?**

Blood loss, hepatic ischemia and the amount of remaining liver.

○   **What palliative treatments are available for the management of unresectable HCC?**

Chemoembolization, injection of alcohol into smaller tumors and cryoablation.

○   *What is the value of PET scanning in the evaluation of patients with colorectal metastases to the liver?*

It may allow identification of additional lesions in the liver or outside of the liver that may render curative resection impossible.

O   **What treatment options are available for hepatic cysts?**

Observation, aspiration, sclerosis, various forms of internal drainage and resection.

O   **What organisms produce hydatid cysts of the liver?**

Echinococcus granulosus and Echinococcus multilocularis.

O   **What is the advantage of a selective shunt over a nonselective shunt?**

A selective shunt will preserve hepatic blood flow and reduce the risk of portosystemic encephalopathy.

O   **What is the first line of therapy for patients with bleeding esophageal varices?**

Endoscopic banding or sclerotherapy.

O   **What is the risk of death from bleeding esophageal varices?**

20 to 50%.

O   **What is the role of propranolol in the management of patients with bleeding esophageal varices?**

It reduces the risk of rebleeding after a first bleed by decreasing the portal pressure.

O   **What arterial supply is shared by the head of the pancreas and the second and third portions of the duodenum, necessitating en bloc resection of the duodenum with lesions of the pancreatic head?**

The inferior pancreaticoduodenal artery, from the superior mesenteric artery, collateralizes with the superior pancreaticoduodenal artery, arising from the gastroduodenal artery.

O   *What is the only pancreatic enzyme secreted in active form?*

Amylase.

O   **What are the most frequent complications following major hepatic resection?**

Hemorrhage and bile leak.

O   **What vessels are contained within the gastrosplenic ligament?**

The short gastrics.

O   **What is the primary pathophysiology in acalculous cholecystitis?**

Gallbladder stasis.

O   **What are the clinical features of hereditary spherocytosis?**

Anemia, reticulocytosis, jaundice and splenomegaly.

O   **What is the most common type of thalassemia in the United States?**

Beta-thalassemia.

O   **What are the indications for splenectomy in a patient with Felty's syndrome?**

Recurrent infections with neutropenia, patients requiring transfusion for anemia, profound thrombocytopenia and intractable leg ulcers.

○   **What is the embryologic origin of the spleen?**

Mesenchymal differentiation in the dorsal mesogastrum.

○   **What are the normal splenic functions?**

Reservoir for circulating platelets, blood filter of old/damaged RBCs, bacteria and particulate antigens, phagocytosis and production of tuftsin, antibodies (especially IgM), opsonins and properdin.

○   **What is the main chemical component of pigment gallstones?**

Calcium bilirubinate.

○   **A 23 year old IV drug abuser presents to the emergency room with fever, chills, splenomegaly and left upper quadrant abdominal tenderness. What is the most likely diagnosis?**

Splenic abscess.

○   **What are the indications for operation in patients with splenic injury?**

Injuries to other intraabdominal organs, increasing peritoneal signs and evidence of continued bleeding.

○   **What is the risk of overwhelming postsplenectomy sepsis in children? In adults?**

0.6% in children and 0.3% in adults.

○   **What are the principle anions in pancreatic juice?**

Bicarbonate and chloride.

○   **What is the anatomic relationship of the uncinate process of the pancreas to the portal vein and superior mesenteric vessels?**

It is posterior.

○   **What cells synthesize somatostatin?**

Delta cells.

○   **What is the embryologic etiology of an annular pancreas?**

Abnormal rotation and fusion of the ventral pancreatic primordium.

○   **What is the significance of the colon cut-off sign?**

It is caused by inflammation of the pancreas, which induces spasm in the adjacent colon.

○   **In what region of the pancreas do most pseudocysts occur?**

The body.

○   **How long does it take for a pseudocyst to mature sufficiently enough for surgical resection?**

4 to 6 weeks (unless the cyst arises during acute pancreatitis, in which case no waiting is necessary).

○   **What is the classic diagnostic (Whipple's) triad for insulinoma?**

Hypoglycemic symptoms produced by fasting, blood glucose less than 50 mg/dl during symptomatic episodes and relief of symptoms with intravenous administration of glucose.

○   **What is Courvoisier's sign and what does its presence suggest?**

It is a distended and palpable gallbladder in a jaundiced patient. It suggests malignant obstruction.

○   **What characteristic finding on ERCP suggests pancreatic cancer?**

Constriction of the pancreatic and bile ducts in the head of the gland (the double duct sign).

○   **Resection of what organs are included in the Whipple procedure?**

The distal stomach, gallbladder, common bile duct, head of the pancreas, duodenum, proximal jejunum and regional lymphatics.

○   **What is the etiology of Zollinger-Ellison syndrome?**

Gastric acid hypersecretion caused by excessive gastrin production.

○   **What percentage of gastrinomas are associated with the MEN-1 syndrome?**

25% (the most common islet cell tumor in MEN-1 syndrome).

○   *What is the typical constellation of symptoms seen in patients with glucagonomas?*

Migratory necrolytic dermatitis, weight loss, stomatitis, hypoaminoacidemia and mild diabetes.

○   **T/F: Cigarette smoking is the most strongly associated risk factor for adenocarcinoma of the pancreas.**

True.

○   **Glycolysis generates how many molecules of ATP for each molecule of glucose?**

37; with 1 molecule utilized for storage.

○   **T/F: The falciform ligament demarcates the right hepatic lobe from the left hepatic lobe.**

False.

○   **When performing complex biliary procedures, where in the hepatoduodenal ligament would you expect to find the common bile duct?**

The duct is most lateral with the hepatic artery medial and the portal vein most posterior.

○   **What is the primary indication for hepatic resection in cirrhotic patients?**

Hepatocellular carcinoma.

○   **In evaluating ascitic fluid obtained from a patient presumed to have SBP, what laboratory findings are expected?**

A WBC count greater than 500/μl with greater than 25% PMNs, a serum albumin:ascitic fluid albumin gradient greater than 1.1 gm/dl, a serum lactic acid level greater than 33 mg/dl or an ascitic fluid pH of less than 7.31.

❍ *What is the treatment of choice for hepatocellular adenomas?*

Surgical excision.

SMALL INTESTINE, COLON, RECTUM AND ANUS PEARLS

Hypochondria is the only disease I haven't got.
Anonymous

○ **What structures are supplied by the superior mesenteric artery (SMA)?**

The cecum, ascending colon and transverse colon.

○ **Where is the SMA in relation to the pancreas?**

Posterior.

○ *Which gut hormone is released from small bowel mucosa after contact with tryptophan and/or fatty acids and results in secretion of enzymes by pancreatic acinar cells?*

Cholecystokinin.

○ **Where is the arc of Riolan?**

Between the left colic artery and the middle colic artery.

○ *Where are bile salts reabsorbed?*

In the ileum.

○ **What is Waldeyer's fascia?**

The dense rectosacral fascia that covers the sacrum and overlying vessels and nerves.

○ *What is the energy source for active sodium transport in the colon?*

Short-chain fatty acids.

○ **What is the most frequent type of colonic motility?**

Mass movements.

○ *What is the strongest component of the small bowel wall?*

The submucosa.

○ **What hormones inhibit colonic motility?**

Glucagon and somatostatin.

○ *What are the most abundant organisms found in the colon?*

Bacteroides and Escherichia coli.

❍   **What signs and symptoms are associated with alkaline gastric reflux?**

Postprandial epigastric pain, nausea, vomiting and gastric biliary reflux.

❍   **A 24 year old female with known peptic ulcer disease (PUD) has been managed adequately with H2 blockers when she finds she has become pregnant. What alterations in her medical therapy should be made?**

Sucralfate is the recommended therapy for PUD in pregnancy, as it has minimal systemic absorption and acceptable healing rates of 80% in 6 weeks.

❍   **What medication is contraindicated in the above patient?**

Misoprostol.

❍   **What are the indications for surgery for patients with PUD?**

Perforation, hemorrhage, obstruction and intractability.

❍   **A 40 year old female presents with nausea, palpatations, epigastric pain and diarrhea within 20 minutes of eating. Her history is significant for a Billroth I procedure for PUD. What is the most likely diagnosis?**

Early dumping syndrome.

❍   **In which region of the colon does volvulus most frequently occur?**

The sigmoid colon.

❍   **What is the etiology of cecal volvulus?**

Anomalous fixation of the right colon to the retroperitoneum.

❍   **Where do colonic diverticula most frequently occur?**

In the sigmoid colon.

❍   **What are the most common presenting symptoms of acute diverticulitis?**

Left lower quadrant abdominal pain, that may radiate to the suprapubic area, left groin or back and alteration in bowel habits (usually constipation).

❍   **An 83 year old nursing home patient with Alzheimer's disease presents with a 24-hour history of severe abdominal distention, without significant pain or tenderness. Abdominal x-rays reveal a large, air-filled right colon. What is the most likely diagnosis?**

Ogilvie's syndrome.

❍   *A 50 year old male presents with his second episode of lower GI bleeding from diverticulosis, localized by colonoscopy to the sigmoid. What is the treatment of choice?*

After controlling the hemorrhage, a sigmoid colectomy should be performed. 25% of patients with initial diverticular bleeding have a recurrence and most patients continue to have recurrences without surgical intervention.

O   **What is the test of choice to confirm the diagnosis of diverticulitis?**

CT scan.

O   **A 55 year old male presents with diverticulitis and significant signs of inflammation. What is the treatment of choice?**

Hospitalization, bowel rest, intravenous fluids and broad-spectrum intravenous antibiotics.

O   **What are the most common complication of diverticulitis?**

Fistula and abscess formation.

O   **Following diverticulitis, what is the most common cause of fistula formation between the sigmoid colon and the urinary bladder?**

Sigmoid carcinoma.

O   **What are the most common causes of massive colonic hemorrhage?**

Diverticulosis and angiodysplasia.

O   **In which region of the colon is angiodysplasia most common?**

The cecum and right colon.

O   **What is the definition of massive lower gastrointestinal hemorrhage?**

Bleeding distal to the ligament of Treitz that requires transfusion of 3 units of blood over 24 hours.

O   **What is the distinct advantage of selective mesenteric angiography for determining the source of colonic hemorrhage?**

Vasopressin can be infused through a specific mesenteric artery to stop the bleeding.

O   **What is the most common cause of ischemic colitis?**

Idiopathic.

O   **What findings on contrast enema suggest the diagnosis of ischemic colitis?**

Submucosal hemorrhage, edema and thumb printing of the involved colonic segment.

O   **What is the most common cause of anal stenosis?**

Scarring after anal surgery.

O   **What is proctalgia fugax?**

Weakened muscle and soft tissue between the rectum and vagina after years of straining to defecate.

O   **What is the anatomic distinction between internal and external hemorrhoids?**

Internal hemorrhoids are above the dentate line, external hemorrhoids are below it.

O   **What is the normal function of hemorrhoidal tissue?**

It protects the underlying muscle during defecation and allows complete closure of the anal canal during rest.

○   **What is a second degree internal hemorrhoid?**

One that is prolapsed but reduces spontaneously.

○   **What are the indications for excisional hemorrhoidectomy?**

1. Large third or fourth degree hemorrhoids which cannot be treated on an out-patient basis.
2. Mixed hemorrhoids with an external endoderm component that is not amenable to ligation.
3. Acutely thrombosed or incarcerated hemorrhoids with severe pain and impending gangrene.

○   **What is the most common complication of excisional hemorrhoidectomy?**

Urinary retention.

○   **T/F: Most anal fissures occur anteriorly.**

False; 90% occur posteriorly in the midline.

○   **A 33 year old male presents with a brief history of severe, burning anal pain during and after bowel movements, accompanied by blood stained toilet paper. What is the most likely diagnosis?**

An anal fissure.

○   *What diagnoses must be entertained if an anal fissure occurs in an unusual location?*

Crohn's disease or tuberculosis.

○   **What percentage of simple anal fissures are amenable to conservative management?**

90%.

○   **What is the treatment of choice for anal fissures that do not respond to conservative therapy?**

Lateral internal sphincterotomy.

○   **Which antibiotics are most frequently implicated in the development of pseudomembranous colitis?**

Clindamycin (most notorious), ampicillin and cephalosporins.

○   **What organism is associated with pseudomembranous colitis?**

C. difficile.

○   *What is the antibiotic of choice for C. difficile colitis?*

Intravenous or oral metronidazole or oral vancomycin (metronidazole contraindicated in pregnancy).

○   **What is the most common protozoon that infects the colon?**

E. histolytica.

○   **Which form of E. histolytica causes infection?**

The cystic form (not the trophozoite).

○   **What is the treatment of choice for E. histolytica?**

Metronidazole and iodoquinol.

○   **Why is 99mTc-pertechnetate used for radionuclide scanning of symptomatic Meckel's diverticula?**

The radioisotope is taken up by heterotopic gastric mucosa within the diverticulum.

○   **T/F: The most common clinical manifestation of Meckel's diverticulum in pediatric patiens is ?**

Bleeding.

○   **What percentage of patients with AIDS develop cytomegalovirus (CMV) colitis?**

90%.

○   **What is the treatment of choice for CMV colitis?**

Dihydroxy-propoxymethyl guanine (DHPG) or gancyclovir.

○   **What is the etiology of Chaga's disease?**

Trypanosoma cruzi.

○   **What are the effects of Chaga's disease on the colon?**

Destruction of Auerbach's myenteric plexus, intramural fibrosis, loss of normal propulsive ability, functional obstruction and proximal megacolon.

○   **What are the contents of the ischiorectal fossa?**

The inferior rectal vessels and lymphatics.

○   **What is the result of abscess formation from cryptoglandular disease with a persistent infected tract?**

Fistula-in-ano.

○   *What is the treatment of Squamous cell Ca of anal canal?*

Nigro protocal: Chemo and RT.

○   *T/F: FAP develop polyps limited to colon.*

False. They may have UGI polyps also so evaluation of duodenum is also needed.

○   *T/F: Familial adenomatous polyposis is autosomal dominant and most pts get cancer by the age of 40 therefore total prophylactic colectomy with mucoproctectomy is recommended.*

True.

○   **What other cancers are associated with lynch II (hereditary non-polyposis colorectal cancer) ?**

Stomach.
Ovary.
Bladder.

○   *Cancers in lynch one are on what side of the colon?*

Usually right sided.

○   *Lynch I and II is associated with what genetic mutation?*

DNA mismatch repair gene.

○   **What are the Amsterdam criteria?**

3 first degree relatives affected over 2 generations.

○   *What is the treatment of Sigmoid volvulous?*

Endoscopic decompression with sigmoidectomy the same hospital admission.

○   **What is the treatment for ileo-anal pouchitis?**

Flagyl and short chain fatty acid enemas.

○   **What is the treatment for pyoderma gangrenosum?**

Dapsone and steroids, avoid operation unless erosion into arterial circulation occurs.

○   **What is the most common manifestation of anal gland infection?**

Perianal abscess.

○   **What is the treatment of choice for a patient with an intersphencteric abscess?**

Internal sphincterotomy.

○   **Why are supralevator abscesses not drained externally or through the ischiorectal fossa?**

They usually do not heal without a diverting colostomy.

○   **What percentage of patients with a perirectal abscess will have a recurrence?**

50%.

○   **What is Goodsall's rule?**

In the treatment of fistula-in-ano, if the anus is transected in a transverse fashion, external openings anterior to the incision will connect with an internal opening by a short, direct fistulous tract.

○   **What is the appropriate management for patients with a horseshoe fistula?**

Incision and drainage of the postanal space and counter drainage of the lateral ischiorectal spaces through separate incisions.

○   **Where is the opening in a high rectovaginal fistula?**

Near the cervix.

○   **What are the most common causes of midrectovaginal fistulas?**

Extension of an undrained ischiorectal abscess, Crohn's disease, surgical excision or fulguration of an anterior rectal tumor, radiation injury and extensive childbirth trauma.

○   **What is the treatment of choice for patients with a midrectovaginal fistula?**

An endorectal advancement flap.

○   **What is a pilonidal cyst?**

A hair-containing sinus or abscess that involves the skin and subcutaneous tissues in the postsacral intergluteal region.

○   *Appendectomy is done revealing carcinoid of the appendix what is the treatment?*
< 2 cm- appendectomy.
>2 cm- R hemicolectomy.

○   *Operation for appendectomy and Crohns' disease is discovered, what is the treatment?*

Appendectomy with appropriate medical management of the Crohn's disease.

○   **What is the appropriate treatment for hidradenitis suppurativa?**

Wide excision, including the indurated overlying skin.

○   **What is the most common cause of perianal pruritis in children?**

Enterobius vermicularis (pinworms).

○   **What is the treatment of choice for pinworms?**

Piperazine citrate.

○   **What is the etiology of lymphogranuloma venereum (LGV)?**

Chlamydia trachomatis.

○   **What is the typical presentation of a patient with chlamydial proctitis?**

Anal pain, pruritis, rectal bleeding or rectal discharge.

○   **What are the secondary lesions of syphilis?**

Condyloma lata.

○   **How is chancroid manifested?**

With soft, multiple lesions that are very painful and friable.

○   **What is the treatment of choice for chancroid?**

Sulfonamides.

○   **What is the treatment of choice for large warts caused by Condylomata acuminata?**

Excision and electrocoagulation.

○   **What is the rate of recurrence of condyloma after local treatment?**

65%.

○   **What layer(s) of the colon is/are affected by ulcerative colitis?**

The mucosal layer only.

○   **What are the extraintestinal manifestations of ulcerative colitis?**

Uveitis, iritis, episcleritis, keratitis, conjunctivitis, peripheral joint disease, arthralgias with progressive edema and erythema, ankylosing spondylitis, sacroiliitis, apthous stomatitis, gingivitis, pyoderma gangrenosum and sclerosing cholangitis.

○   **Which of the inflammatory bowel diseases (IBDs) has a continuous distribution in the colon?**

Ulcerative colitis.

○   **T/F: TPN is superior to enteral diets in achieving remission of small intestinal Crohn's disease.**

False.

○   **What percentage of patients with Crohn's disease have rectal involvement?**

50%.

○   **What is the most frequent gastrointestinal site of Crohn's disease?**

The ileocecal region, which accounts for approximately 50% of cases.

○   **What colonoscopic findings are associated with Crohn's disease?**

Linear ulcerations, cobble-stoning, asymmetric involvement, skip lesions and apthous ulcers.

○   **In which of the IBDs are strictures most common?**

Crohn's disease.

○   **What are the morphologic characteristics of moderately severe ulcerative colitis?**

Progression of mucosal disease with purulent discharge, diffuse ulceration and bleeding and formation of pseudopolyps.

○   **What are the indications for surgery in patients with ulcerative colitis?**

Active disease unresponsive to medical management, risk of cancer and severe hemorrhage.

○   **What is the increased risk of colon cancer related to in patients with ulcerative colitis?**

The extent of mucosal involvement and the duration of the disease.

○   **What are the indications for surgery in patients with Crohn's disease?**

Internal fistulas and abscesses, intestinal obstruction, toxic megacolon and poor response to medical therapy.

○   *What region of the colon is usually involved with Type I Lynch syndrome?*

The proximal colon.

○   **What extraintestinal manifestations are associated with familial adenomatous polyposis (FAP)?**

Epidermoid cysts, dermoid tumors of the abdomen, osteomas and brain tumors (usually gliomas and medulloblastomas).

O   *What percentage of patients with untreated FAP develop colon cancer?*

100%.

O   **When should screening colonoscopy be initiated for family members of patients with FAP?**

At 10 years of age.

O   **What is the treatment of choice for patients with FAP and greater than 50 rectal polyps?**

Total proctocolectomy, ileoanal pouch anastamosis and an ileal reservoir.

O   **What is the risk of developing colorectal carcinoma in a patient with a first-degree relative that has colorectal carcinoma?**

3 to 9 times that of the normal population.

O   **What is the most accurate method of detecting polyps greater than 1 cm?**

Colonoscopy.

O   **Patients with which IBD have the greatest incidence of developing colon carcinoma?**

Those with ulcerative colitis.

O   **What is the inheritance pattern of Peutz-Jeghers syndrome?**

Autosomal dominant.

O   **What is bacterial translocation?**

Passage of viable bacteria from the intact gastrointestinal tract lumen to mesenteric lymph nodes and possibly the liver. Small intestinal integrity is impaired as a result of a variety of systemic injuries.

O   **How can the incidence of bacterial translocation be decreased?**

By enteral feeding.

O   **What is the most common cause of gastrointestinal bleeding in childhood?**

Meckles diverticulum.

O   **What is the increased risk of cancer in patients with a single juvenile polyp?**

None.

O   **What is the most common type of adenomatous colonic polyp?**

Tubular adenoma (65 to 80%).

O   **T/F: Polypectomy decreases the risk of colon cancer.**

True.

❍   **What percentage of patients with colorectal carcinoma have a synchronous polyp?**

30%.

❍   **What preoperative testing should be done prior to colon resection for carcinoma?**

Chest x-ray, CT scan of the abdomen, liver function tests and a serum CEA level.

❍   **What is the procedure of choice for a patient with carcinoma in the right colon?**

A right hemicolectomy, including 10 cm of terminal ileum, with ligation of the ileocolic artery, right colic artery and the right branch of the middle colic artery.

❍   **What margins of resection are required for colon carcinoma?**

5 cm is ideal, however, 2 cm may be adequate.

❍   **What factors are related to prognosis for patients with colon carcinoma?**

Depth of invasion, lymph node involvement and presence or absence of distant metastases.

❍   **What is the 5-year survival for patients with Stage II colon carcinoma?**

60 to 80%.

❍   **What is the most influential prognostic indicator of rectal carcinoma?**

Lymph node involvement.

❍   **What is the procedure of choice for patients with rectal carcinoma in whom the sphincter mechanism cannot be preserved?**

Abdominal perineal resection (APR).

❍   **A 38 year old female presents with colonic perforation, secondary to toxic megacolon associated with ulcerative colitis. What is the appropriate surgical procedure?**

Abdominal colectomy with Hartmann closure of the rectum.

❍   **If continuity can be restored without tension and without sacrificing the blood supply, what procedure should be performed for patients with rectal carcinoma?**

A low anterior resection (LAR).

❍   **What is the appropriate operation for gallstone ileus?**

Identification of the impacted gallstone in the small bowel followed by proximal enterotomy, with retrieval of the gallstone. Cholecystectomy should not be performed at the initial operation if the patient is acutely ill or exhibiting signs of sepsis.

❍   **What is the overall incidence of clinically evident ischemic colitis following aortic reconstruction?**

1 to 2%.

❍   **What is the most significant factor related to improved outcome for ischemic colitis?**

Early diagnosis.

❍ *What is the treatment of choice for acute superior mesenteric artery (SMA) thrombosis?*

Mesenteric revascularization and resection of non-viable bowel, followed by a second-look laparotomy the next day.

❍ **What are the angiographic criteria for non-occlusive mesenteric ischemia?**

Narrowing at the origins of major SMA branches, irregularities of further branches with alternating dilation and constriction, spasm of peripheral arcades and impaired filling of intramural vessels.

❍ **What is the most frequent angiographic finding of an SMA embolism?**

A meniscus sign within the artery, 3 to 8 cm. from its origin, where proximal jejunal branches fill promptly (distal jejunal, ileal and colic branches do not fill).

❍ **What are the classic symptoms of chronic mesenteric ischemia?**

Postprandial pain, weight loss and fear of food. Occasionally, bloody diarrhea may be present.

❍ **What is primary mesenteric venous thrombosis?**

Spontaneous occlusion of the mesenteric veins, without trauma or co-existing hematologic, liver or cardiac disease.

❍ **Which recreational drug has been associated with ischemic colitis?**

Cocaine.

❍ **How long should patients who have had an episode of acute mesenteric venous thrombosis and do not have a contraindication to anticoagulation, be anticoagulated?**

Life-long.

❍ **What is the gender ratio for patients with celiac compression syndrome?**

Females 4:1.

❍ **What peak systolic velocity criteria, by duplex scanning of the SMA, is suggestive of chronic mesenteric ischemia?**

275 cm/sec.

❍ **What is the mortality rate of acute intestinal ischemia once intestinal infarction occurs?**

70 to 90%.

❍ **Manipulation of the aortic arch during cardiac surgery may cause mesenteric ischemia by what phenomenon?**

Cholesterol immobilization with embolization.

❍ **What is the single most important issue in managing patients with short gut syndrome following massive bowel infarction?**

Optimizing nutritional status.

❍   **In a patient with intestinal ischemia, when should the decision to perform a second look laparotomy be made?**

At the initial operation, prior to closing the abdomen.

❍   **What is the conduit of choice during mesenteric revascularization?**

The saphanous vein.

❍   **What is the initial success rate of percutaneous transluminal angioplasty (PTA) for chronic mesenteric ischemia?**

80 to 90%.

❍   **What is a surgical alternative to mesenteric revascularization for chronic mesenteric ischemia?**

Transaortic splanchnic endarterectomy.

❍   **What is the most common splanchnic artery aneurysm?**

Splenic artery aneurysm.

❍   **What classification of drugs are often associated with non-occlusive mesenteric ischemia?**

Vasopressor and alpha-adrenergic agonists.

❍   **What are the most important predictors of success in patients surgically treated for celiac compression syndrome?**

A classic history of postprandial pain, weight loss and decreased food intake and significant stenosis of the celiac axis. Negative clinical response is correlated with atypical symptoms.

❍   **What percentage of patients with intestinal ischemia have mesenteric venous thrombosis as the etiology?**

5 to 15%.

❍   **What is the potential sequelae of ischemic colitis when it involves the muscular layer and fibrosis occurs?**

Late stricture formation.

❍   **What clinical scenarios are produced by spontaneous dissection of a mesenteric artery?**

Intraabdominal hemorrhage and bowel ischemia.

❍   **What antibodies may be present in patients with systemic lupus erythematosus, who develop intestinal ischemia?**

Anticardiolipin and anitphospolipid antibodies.

❍   **Which visceral aneurysms may arise as a complication of pancreatitis?**

Pancreaticoduodenal and gastroduodenal artery aneurysms.

❍   **Acute mesenteric ischemia accounts for what percentage of the intraabdominal complications of cardiopulmonary bypass?**

Up to 33%.

❍   **What phenomenon leads to a sequence of events that, paradoxically, leads to tissue damage in patients with mesenteric ischemia?**

Reperfusion injury.

❍   **What two essential features of the management of mesenteric ischemia have significantly improved survival?**

Extensive use of arteriography and transcatheter intraarterial papaverine.

❍   *The migrating myoelectric complex (MMC), which occurs during the interdigestive period in the small intestine, is primarily under neurologic and humeral control via which intestinal hormone?*

Motilin.

❍   *Which gut hormone functions as a negative control for the release of virtually all other intestinal hormones?*

Somatostatin.

❍   **Which cells in the intestinal lumen are responsible for antigen uptake and transport to underlying lymphoid nodules?**

M cells.

❍   **What is the most frequent urologic complication of ileocolic Crohn's disease?**

Ureteral obstruction.

❍   **T/F: Resection margins for small intestinal Crohn's disease should be proven histologically negative by frozen section.**

False.

❍   **What is the appropriate operative approach for patients with Crohn's disease who develop non-healing, symptomatic ileosigmoid fistulas?**

Resection of the diseased terminal ileum and oversewing of the sigmoid colon, if grossly uninvolved with Crohn's disease.

❍   **Primary tubercular infection of the terminal ileum is due to which strain?**

The bovine strain of Mycobacterium, resulting from ingestion of infected milk.

❍   **Secondary infection of the terminal ileum by tuberculosis is due to which strain?**

The human strain of Mycobacterium tuberculosis, secondary to swallowing of bacilli by patients with active pulmonary disease.

❍   **What are the most common indications for surgery for patients with small bowel leiomyomas?**

Bleeding and obstruction.

❍   **What is the 5-year survival rate following curative resection of adenocarcinoma of the jejunum or ileum?**

Less than 20%.

○   *An elevated level of what chemical compounds is associated with malignant carcinoid syndrome?*

5-hydroxyindoleacetic acid (5-HIAA) and vanillylmandelic acid (VMA).

○   **What is the safest and most reliable provocative test for the diagnosis of malignant carcinoid syndrome?**

The pentagastrin test.

○   **What is the surgical management for patients with duodenal diverticula imbedded deep within the head of the pancreas?**

Lateral duodenotomy, followed by invagination of the diverticulum into the lumen, excision of the diverticulum and closure of both walls.

○   **Where do the majority of duodenal malignancies occur?**

In the periampullary region.

○   **What factors are associated with failure of spontaneous closure of small bowel fistulas?**

Disruption of greater than 50% of intestinal continuity, active granulomatous disease, cancer or radiation enteritis in the segment, distal bowel obstruction, foreign body, undrained abscess in relation to the fistula and epithelialization of the tract.

○   **In low-output small bowel fistulas, conservative therapy should be continued for what period of time?**

Up to 6 weeks.

○   **What percentage of adults with small bowel intussusception do not have an associated underlying pathologic process?**

10%.

○   **What percentage of adults with intussusception have an underlying tumor?**

Over 65% are associated with benign or malignant tumors.

○   *Patients with Crohn's disease, who have extensive terminal ileal disease or who have had previous ileal resections, are prone to what type of kidney stones?*

Urate and oxalate stones.

○   **What is the most frequent location for villous adenomas in the small intestine?**

The duodenum.

○   **What is the 5-year survival after curative resection for localized leiomyosarcoma of the small intestine?**

40 to 50%.

○   **Immunoproliferative small intestinal disease (IPSID), which occurs in the Mediterranean Basin, is associated with what abnormality?**

Increase in the IgA heavy chain fragment in serum, secondary to diffuse infiltration of plasma cytoid lymphoma cells within the intestinal wall.

O   **What is the appropriate therapy for localized primary lymphoma of the small intestine?**

Wide resection with en bloc lymphadenectomy.

O   **What is the most common source of hematogenously spread malignancy to the small intestine?**

Malignant melanoma.

O   *A 65 year old female presents with mild abdominal distention, nausea and vomiting. A KUB indicates pneumobilia and paucity of air in the colon. What is the most likely diagnosis?*

Gallstone ileus, due to a fistulous communication between the gallbladder and the duodenum. Stones greater than 2.5 cm may become obstructed at the ileocecal valve.

O   *A 50 year old male with chronic atrial fibrillation but no prior surgical history presents with 24 hours of nausea and vomiting, moderate abdominal tenderness and abdominal distention. The KUB shows dilated loops of small bowel with multiple air fluid levels and the PT is 75. What is the treatment of choice?*

Nasogastric decompression, administration of vitamin K and discontinuation of anticoagulation.

O   *T/F: A right hemicolectomy is the treatment of choice for a patient with a noninvasive 1.9 cm appendiceal carcinoid at the mid-portion of the appendix.*

False. If the margins are negative, an appendectomy may be done for a carcinoid tumor at this site. If the carcinoid is greater than 2 cm, invasive or involves the base, a hemicolectomy should be performed.

O   **What factors contribute to development of the blind loop syndrome?**

Absence of the gastric acidic barrier, with increased introduction of bacteria to the small bowel, abnormal communication between the stomach and the intestine, anatomic etiologies and motility disorders.

O   **What is the treatment for patients with blind loop syndrome?**

Appropriate antibiotic therapy frequently results in relief of symptoms within 1 week. The underlying etiology should be addressed if symptoms recur.

O   **A 35 year old male with intractable ulcer disease has severe scarring in the peripyloric region. What type of pyloroplasty is most appropriate after truncal vagotomy?**

A Jaboulay pyloroplasty. It includes a gastroduodenostomy while bypassing the pylorus.

O   **What is involved in a Finney pyloroplasty?**

A longitudinal incision in the pyloric musculature, from the gastric antrum to the duodenum and a gastroduodenostomy.

O   **What is the Heineke-Mikulizc procedure?**

A longitudinal incision of the pylorus that is closed transversely.

O   **What conservative measures are appropriate for alkaline reflux gastritis?**

H2-blockers, antacids, bile chelators and dietary changes.

O   **What is the treatment of choice for alkaline reflux gastritis if conservative measures fail?**

Creation of a Roux-en-Y anastomosis with a 50 to 60 cm Roux limb.

O   **Which segment of the GI tract is the most common location for a Kaposi's sarcoma?**

The duodenum.

O   **A 39 year old female presents with hypokalemia, a hypochloremic metabolic acidosis and copious diarrhea. A polyp is found on colonoscopy. What is the most likely diagnosis?**

A villous adenoma.

INTRAABDOMINAL INFECTIONS AND SURGICAL COMPLICATIONS PEARLS

The abdomen is the reason why man does not easily take himself for a god.
Freidrich Nietzsche

○ **What is the most common source of bacteria in postoperative surgical infections?**

The patient.

○ **What perioperative factors are associated with an increased risk of postoperative wound infection?**

Long preoperative hospitalization, no preoperative shower, early shaving of the operative site, hair removal and prior antibiotic therapy.

○ **What factors can impair phagocytosis of bacteria?**

Bacterial encapsulation, uremia, prematurity, leukemia and hyperglycemia.

○ **Which antibiotic agents are bacteriostatic?**

Chloramphenicol, clindamycin, erythromycin, sulfonamides, tetracyclines and trimethoprim.

○ **Why are iodine solutions superior to chlorhexidine as a surgical antiseptic?**

Chlorhexidine is not effective against viruses and fungi.

○ ***What is the toxic portion of the endotoxin lipopolysaccharide protein complex?***

Lipid A.

○ ***What is the mechanism of action of quinolones?***

They inhibit DNA gyrase, which is needed to package DNA into dividing bacteria.

○ **What is the best time to begin prophylactic antibiotic therapy for elective surgery?**

1 hour prior to the operation.

○ **What is the incidence of wound infections in clean, clean contaminated, contaminated and dirty cases?**

Less than 2%, 10%, 20% and 40%, respectively.

○ **T/F: Closed suction drainage decreases the incidence of wound infection in clean cases.**

False.

❍   **What is the most common cause of fascial dehiscence other than poor surgical technique?**

Intraabdominal sepsis.

❍   **In patients with postoperative pneumonia, empiric monotherapy should cover which organisms?**

Gram negative organisms.

❍   **What factors suggest failure or recurrence following percutaneous intraabdominal abscess drainage?**

Persistent low grade fevers, persistent leukocytosis and continued or increased volume of drainage.

❍   **Which intraabdominal abscesses respond poorly to percutaneous drainage?**

Subphrenic and pancreatic abscesses.

❍   **A 50 year old female alcoholic is admitted to the hospital with the diagnosis of acute pancreatitis. She is readmitted 2 weeks after discharge with complaints of abdominal pain and fever. Laboratory evaluation reveals a decreased hematocrit and an increased WBC count. What is the most likely diagnosis?**

A pancreatic abscess.

❍   **What is abdominal compartment syndrome?**

Increased pressure within the confined anatomical space of the abdomen that may impair end-organ perfusion and physiologic function.

❍   **How is intraabdominal pressure measured?**

The direct method requires placement of a cannula into the peritoneal cavity. Indirect methods include measurement of inferior vena cava pressure, gastric pressure or urinary bladder pressure.

❍   **What is the treatment of choice for patients with a perforation of the cervical esophagus?**

Cervical exploration, drainage of the superior mediastinum and antibiotics.

❍   **What is the mortality rate for patients with leaking ascites following major surgery? What is the appropriate treatment?**

As high as 60%; return to the operating room for repair of fascial dehiscence.

❍   **A 40 year old Chinese male presents with jaundice, high fever and rigors. What organism will most likely be detected?**

Opisthorchiasis (Clonorchis) sinesis.

❍   *48 hours postoperatively, a patient develops severe pain in his midline wound, skin bullae, crepitus, irregular blanching at the would margins and a fever of 104° F. What diagnosis must be considered?*

Clostridial gas gangrene.

❍   **A 40 year old female presents with a common bile duct obstruction. Records show that she had previously undergone a cholecystectomy with a choledochoduodenostomy. Evaluation reveals a retained stone in the common bile duct (CBD). What error was made by the initial surgeon?**

He did not dilate the CBD prior to performing the choledochoduodenostomy.

○   **What is the proper treatment for iatrogenic transection of the CBD?**

End-to-end anastamosis (EEA) over a T-tube stent.

○   **What factors increase mortality in patients with esophageal perforation?**

Delay in diagnosis and treatment, severe underlying esophageal disease, need for a major extirpative procedure and an intrathoracic site of perforation.

○   **What is the average mortality rate from acute esophageal variceal bleeding?**

20 to 25%.

○   **A 25 year old multiple trauma patient develops bright red upper gastrointestinal bleeding on SICU day 6. What is the first step in management?**

Upper endoscopy to identify the source of bleeding.

○   **A postoperative patient with coffee ground nasogastric aspirates is found to have diffuse gastritis on upper endoscopy. What is the most appropriate initial therapy?**

Medical treatment with antacids, H2-blockers or sucralfate and correction of any coagulation defects.

○   **T/F: Anaphylactic shock may follow intraperitoneal rupture of a hydatid cyst.**

True.

○   **Which structure is most commonly injured if the triangle of Calot is not identified during cholecystectomy?**

The right hepatic artery.

○   **A 69 year old male develops sudden onset of fever, chills, tachycardia and hypotension 4 days following placement of a percutaneous endoscopic gastrostomy (PEG) tube. Physical examination reveals abdominal distension and plain abdominal films show a large amount of free air. What is the most likely diagnosis?**

Gastric leakage secondary to necrosis.

○   **What is the drug of choice for patients with peritonitis caused by Bacteroides fragilis?**

Metronidazole.

○   **What is the most likely diagnosis in a 45 year old female with acute cholecystitis, a WBC count of 30,000/mm3 and evidence of intramural gas in the gallbladder?**

An emphysematous gallbladder.

○   **T/F: The treatment of choice for a patient with an amebic liver abscess is surgical drainage.**

False, metronidazole is Tx.

○   **What is the most common cause of early small bowel obstructions?**

Small bowel adhesions.

❍   *A 60 year old female presents with severe weight loss and steatorrhea following extensive small bowel resection. What is the most common cause of her symptoms?*

Resection of the ileum with resultant insufficient bile salt absorption.

❍   **What is the incidence of early small bowel obstruction (within 30 days) following laparotomy?**

1 to 3%.

❍   **A 30 year old female develops a small bowel obstruction six days after exploratory laparotomy for a gun shot wound to the abdomen. What is the treatment of choice?**

Nasogastric decompression, unless there are signs of ischemia or strangulation.

❍   **What is the most feared complication of duodenal surgery?**

A duodenal fistula with intraabdominal sepsis.

❍   *What is the most common complication in a patient who received postoperative radiation therapy following radical prostatectomy?*

Rectal bleeding. Tx is formic acid enema.

❍   **What is the initial therapy for clostridium difficile colitis?**

Oral metronidazole or vancomycin. For patients with severe ileus, intravenous metronidazole and vancomycin enemas may have some merit.

❍   **What is the appropriate surgical therapy for toxic clostridium difficile colitis?**

Total colectomy and end-ileostomy.

❍   **A 30 year old female was treated in India for intestinal obstruction secondary to tuberculosis. What is the next step in treatment?**

A full course of antituberculous antibiotics.

❍   **What factors increase the risk of complications after major surgery in a patient with liver cirrhosis?**

Encephalopathy, hypoalbuminemia, malnutrition, prolonged PT and performance of a partial hepatectomy.

❍   **What is the appropriate workup for patients with lower gastrointestinal bleeding?**

Localization of the bleeding site with a bleeding scan or angiography.

❍   *Why is angiographic embolization a poor choice for treatment of patients with lower gastrointestinal bleeding?*

The bleeding vessels are end-arteries, thus, embolization would likely cause necrosis.

❍   **What two classes of mediators are responsible for the hemodynamic, metabolic and immune responses to bacteremia?**

Humoral mediators (e.g., catecholamines, glucocorticoids, glucagon) and cytokines.

❍   **Which cytokines are known to be involved in the cellular response to infection?**

TNF, IL-1, IL-2, IL-6 and interferon-gamma.

○ **T/F: Lactation should be discontinued in women with mastitis.**

False. Breast feeding can continue with both breasts unless suppuration is significant.

○ **What bacteria is commonly reported as the sole cause of nonclostridial necrotizing soft tissue infection?**

Beta-hemolytic streptococcus.

○ *What is the best predictor for the development of spontaneous bacterial peritonitis (SBP) in cirrhotic patients?*

The amount of protein in the ascitic fluid. Patients with an ascitic fluid protein concentration of 1 gm/dl are 10 times more likely to develop SBP than those with a level of less than 1g/dl.

○ **Which abscesses are associated with a high failure rate with percutaneous CT guided drainage?**

Pancreatic abscess, abscesses following splenectomy and multiloculated abscesses.

○ **What is the treatment of choice for patients with acute, progressive saphenous thrombophlebitis of the upper thigh?**

Ligation of the greater saphenous vein at the saphenofemoral junction and excision of the thrombosed vein.

○ **What is the difference between pyogenic and tuberculous osteomyelitis of the spine?**

Pyogenic osteomyelitis does not usually result in collapse of the vertebral bodies, tuberculous osteomyelitis does.

○ **What is the initial treatment for patients with lung abscesses?**

Culture of the sputum, appropriate antibiotics and regular bronchoscopy to maintain drainage.

○ **What is the best way to drain a pelvic abscess?**

Through the rectum or vagina.

○ **What organisms are most commonly associated with peritonitis in patients receiving peritoneal dialysis?**

S. aureus and S. epidermidis.

○ *What characteristic is common to clavulanate, sulbactam and tazobactam?*

They are all beta-lactamase inhibitors.

○ **T/F: The dose of metronidazole must be modified for patients with significant liver disease.**

True.

○ **How long should antibiotics be continued in a patient with penetrating abdominal trauma and multiple organ injuries?**

Antibiotics limited to the perioperative period (12 to 24 hours) is adequate provided it was started preoperatively (within 3 to 4 hours of injury).

○   **What antibiotics may be used to treat Clostiridial Perfringes if the patient is penicillin-allergic?**

Cloramphenicol, tetracycline, clindamycin or erythromycin.

○   **What is the significance of candida endophthalmitis?**

It is usually diagnostic of hematogenous infection and may lead to blindness if left untreated.

○   **Under which specific situations would Fluconazole be equivalent to Amphotericin B in the treatment of patients with candidemia?**

In patients who are not severely immunocompromised.

○   **Which pulmonary fungal infection can lead to severe central nervous system disease?**

Cryptococcosis.

○   **What constitutes adequate tetanus immunization for an adult?**

3 injections of toxoid followed by a routine booster of adsorbed toxoid every 10 years.

○   **What is the treatment for a patient with tetanus?**

Excision and debridement of the wound, control of convulsions, antibiotics and 3000 to 6000 units of human tetanus immune globulin.

○   **What is the worst prognostic sign for a patient with a pyogenic liver abscess?**

Multiple abscesses.

○   **What is the significance of a hepatic defect in a patient treated with metronidazole for an amebic liver abscess?**

None. The defect may persist for many months in the cured patient. Operative or percutaneous drainage is rarely indicated except for secondary bacterial complications or failure to respond to metronidazole.

○   **What is the significance of patients who test positive for HBeAg?**

They are one million times more infective than those that are positive for HBsAg only.

○   **What is the latency period for developing antibodies to hepatitis C?**

Up to 4 months.

○   **Which body fluids were involved in all reported HIV seroconversions in health care workers?**

Blood and sanguinous fluids.

○   **What might be the result of cytomegalovirus or cryptosporidial infection of the bile ducts in HIV patients?**

Papillary stenosis or sclerosing cholangitis.

○   **What is the latency period for seroconversion following exposure to the HIV virus?**

6 to 12 months.

❍ **How does the operative mortality and morbidity for elective or emergency abdominal operations in HIV infected, asymptomatic patients compare to that for uninfected patients?**

It is comparable.

❍ **How does the operative mortality and morbidity for elective or emergency abdominal operations in patients with AIDS compare to that for uninfected patients?**

It is slightly higher in elective surgery and significantly higher in emergency surgery.

ABDOMINAL WALL, OMENTUM, MESENTARY AND RETROPERITONEUM PEARLS

The young physician starts life with twenty drugs for each disease.
The old physician ends life with one drug for twenty diseases.
William Osler

○ **Where do the lymphatics of the lower half of the abdominal wall drain?**

To the inguinal nodes, then to the iliac nodes.

○ **What is the most common cause of a rectus sheath hematoma?**

Rupture of the epigastric artery or vein secondary to trauma.

○ **What is the typical presentation of a patient with a rectus sheath hematoma?**

Severe abdominal pain exacerbated by movement, tenderness over the rectus sheath and voluntary guarding.

○ **What structures define the semicircular line?**

The lower edge of the posterior sheath (3 to 6 cm below the umbilicus).

○ **What is the blood supply to the rectus abdominus muscle?**

The superior and inferior epigastric arteries.

○ **What is the composition of the posterior rectus sheath below the linea semicircularis?**

The transversalis fascia.

○ **What is the most common solid omental tumor?**

Metastatic carcinoma.

○ **What is the usual presentation of a small omental cyst?**

An incidental finding at laparotomy.

○ **What is the most common etiology of retroperitoneal fibrosis?**

Idiopathic.

○ **T/F: Typhoid fever is associated with rectus sheath hematomas.**

True.

❍   *T/F: A spigelian hernia is easy to diagnose and not a true surgical hernia.*
False as they are deep to external oblique through the linea semilunaris and inferior to the linea semi-circularis.

❍   **What is the appropriate treatment for patients with an expanding rectus sheath hematoma?**

Evacuation and closure without drains.

❍   **What diagnostic findings are associated with retroperitoneal fibrosis on intravenous pyelography (IVP)?**

Median deviation of the ureter, hydroureteronephrosis and extrinsic ureteral compression.

❍   **What is the function of the mesentery?**

It serves primarily as a suspensory ligament of the jejunum and ileum.

❍   **What vessels run within the transverse mesocolon?**

Branches of the middle colic artery and accompanying vein.

❍   **Radiation therapy for desmoid tumors is very effective for local control. Why does this modality play only a limited role in treatment?**

The radiation dose required, 60 Gy, risks major damage to adjacent structures.

❍   **What are the most common malignant tumors of the mesentery?**

Liposarcoma, lymphoma, leiomyosarcoma.

❍   **What is the most common cause of acute occlusion of the superior mesenteric artery (SMA)?**

Emboli (usually from the heart).

❍   **What are the goals of treatment for patients with retroperitoneal fibrosis?**

Identification and management of potential causative agents, relief of ureteral obstruction and reversal of the inflammatory-fibrotic process.

❍   **What percentage of patients with retroperitoneal fibrosis develop recurrent ureteral obstruction?**

90%.

❍   **What are the clinical characteristics of mesenteric lymphadenitis?**

Vague, migratory abdominal pain that is usually self-limiting.

❍   **Which visceral artery is most frequently affected by aneurysms?**

The splenic artery.

❍   **What are the most common non-visceral malignant tumors of the retroperitoneum?**

Lymphoma, liposarcoma and fibrosarcoma.

❍   **What is the most common cause of splanchnic artery aneurysms?**

Arteriosclerosis.

O   **What is the predominant physical finding in patients with a retroperitoneal tumor?**

A palpable abdominal mass.

O   **What is the blood supply to the anterior abdominal wall?**

The superior and inferior epigastric arteries, the lower intercostal arteries and the circumflex iliac arteries.

ADRENAL, PITUITARY AND HYPOTHALAMUS PEARLS

The man who makes no mistakes does not usually make anything.
Edward John Phelps

○   **What zone of the adrenal gland is spared in autoimmune adrenal disease?**

The medulla.

○   **Secretion of which adrenal hormone is not impaired by secondary adrenal insufficiency?**

Aldosterone.

○   **What is the most common cause of chronic primary adrenal insufficiency (Addison's Disease)?**

Autoimmune disease.

○   **What are the most common causes of acute secondary adrenal insufficiency?**

Sheehan's Syndrome (postpartum pituitary necrosis), bleeding into a pituitary macroadenoma and head trauma.

○   **What diseases produce a slow, insidious progression to primary adrenal insufficiency?**

Autoimmune diseases, tuberculosis, systemic fungal infections, CMV, Kaposi's sarcoma, metastatic carcinoma and lymphoma.

○   **T/F: Orthostatic hypotension and electrolyte abnormalities are more common in primary adrenal insufficiency than in secondary adrenal insufficiency.**

True.

○   **What does the posterior pituitary secrete?**

ADH and Oxytocin.

○   **What does the anterior pituitary secrete?**

GH, ACTH, TSH, LH, FSH, Prolactin.

○   *What vision changes will lead one to suspect a pituitary mass?*

Bilateral hemianopsia.

○   **What are the most specific signs of primary adrenal insufficiency?**

Hyperpigmentation of the skin and mucosal membranes, seen with increased ACTH secretion.

O   **What therapy should be instituted prior to obtaining the results of an adrenal corticotropin hormone (ACTH) stimulation test in a critically ill patient?**

An empiric stress dose of dexamethasone.

O   **How can the ACTH stimulation test be normal in secondary adrenal insufficiency?**

If the gland has not yet atrophied, it retains the ability to be stimulated.

O   **What is the basis of the insulin-induced hypoglycemia test for patients with secondary adrenal insufficiency?**

Hypoglycemia induced by 0.1 units of insulin/kg stimulates the entire hypothalamus-hypophyseal-adrenal axis (HPA) and the sympathetic nervous system. Plasma cortisol levels should exceed 20 g/dl.

O   **What are the contraindications to the insulin-induced hypoglycemia test?**

Patients with cardiac disease and those with a history of seizures.

O   **What is the short metyrapone test?**

Metyrapone inhibits adrenal 11-hydroxylase. Normally the cortisol precursor, 11-deoxycortisol, increases to at least 7 g/dl. This is in response to the decreased production of cortisol and loss of the negative feedback of cortisol to the HPA axis, hence, stimulation of ACTH. This is indicative of secondary adrenal insufficiency only in the setting of a previously measured cortisol level of 8 g/dl.

O   **After an endocrinolgic diagnosis has been established by hormonal studies, what is the radiologic study of choice to assess for a pituitary or hypothalamic tumor?**

MRI with analysis of the sagittal and coronal sections. A CT scan can be helpful if bony invasion is suspected.

O   **What is the emergent steroid replacement for patients with adrenal insufficiency?**

50 to 100 mg of intravenous hydrocortisone every 8 hours.

O   **What patients should receive fluorocortisone?**

Those with primary adrenal insufficiency.

O   **What is the characteristic hemodynamic pattern of adrenal insufficiency?**

Decreased systemic vascular resistance (SVR) and, to a lesser degree, decreased cardiac contractility.

O   **When do the serum corticotropin and cortisol concentrations return to normal following routing surgery?**

Within 24 to 28 hours.

O   **What drugs can impair cortisol synthesis in the critically ill patient?**

Ketoconazole, etomidate and aminoglutethimide.

O   **T/F: Corticosteroids are effective in the treatment of septic shock.**

False.

O   **Randomized prospective trials have shown a benefit from corticosteroids in what disease states?**

Bacterial meningitis, acute spinal injury, typhoid fever, Pneumocystis carinii pneumonia and, possibly, in the treatment of the fibroproliferative phase of adult/acute respiratory distress syndrome (ARDS).

❍ **What diagnostic test is the best predictor of adrenal adequacy in patients previously receiving steroids, who are scheduled for surgery?**

The peak cortisol level after administration of corticotropin.

❍ **What are the adverse effects of excessive cortisol dosing for high stress situations?**

The catabolic effects on muscle, impaired wound healing, inhibition of insulin and the anti-inflammatory effect on active infection.

❍ **How much cortisol is produced each day in patients undergoing minor and major surgery?**

50 mg and 75 to 100 mg, respectively.

❍ **What are the current recommendations for stress doses of cortisol in patients with suspected adrenal insufficiency?**

Minor stress, 25 mg/day; moderate stress, 50 to 75 mg/day and major stress, 100 to 150 mg/day.

❍ **What is the flow phase of the metabolic response to stress?**

It occurs approximately 24 hours after injury and is characterized by a rise in cardiac output, temperature, oxygen consumption and serum insulin levels.

❍ *A 45 year old male develops hypotension and lethargy and has a hemoglobin of 12 gm/dl and a blood glucose of 34 mg/dl 24 hours after colectomy. His history is significant for a renal transplant 3 years ago. What is the most likely diagnosis?*

Addisonian crisis.

❍ **What inhibits growth hormone (GH) secretion?**

Somatostatin.

❍ **T/F: Insulin-like growth factor (IGF-1) is decreased during periods of injury or sepsis.**

True.

❍ **What are the effects of administering GH to patients during periods of stress?**

It increases metabolic rate, fat oxidation and protein synthesis.

❍ **Where does aldosterone exert its primary effect?**

On the distal tubules and collecting ducts of the kidney.

❍ *What is the effect of aldosterone on the kidney?*

It increases the absorption of sodium from the urine in exchange for potassium, thereby aiding in water retention and restoring intravascular volume.

❍ **What are the metabolic effects of catecholamines during periods of stress?**

Increased glycogenolysis, gluconeogenesis, lipolysis and ketogenesis and inhibition of insulin use in peripheral tissues.

O   **What are the beneficial effects of cortisol on cell membranes during times of stress?**

It acts as a cell membrane stabilizer.

O   *What are the functions of angiotensin II?*

Vasoconstriction, cardiac stimulation and stimulation of ADH, aldosterone and thirst.

O   **What is the effect of cortisol, epinephrine and glucagon on protein metabolism?**

They all increase excretion of urinary nitrogen.

O   **What is the blood supply to the posterior lobe of the pituitary gland?**

The inferior hypophyseal artery, a branch from the carotid artery.

O   **Why does the female pituitary gland increase in size by about 10% during pregnancy?**

Hypertrophy of prolactin secreting cells.

O   **What significant problem may occur in individuals in whom the diaphragma sella does not closely surround the pituitary stalk?**

Pituitary tumors may extend superiorly.

O   **What stimuli cause release of ADH (vasopressin)?**

Plasma osmolality greater than 285 mOsm/l, decreased circulating blood volume, catecholamines, the renin-angiotensin system and opiates.

O   **What inhibits release of leutinizing hormone (LH) in the adult male?**

Androgens synthesized by the testes.

O   **What is the function of follicle stimulating hormone (FSH) in the adult female?**

It stimulates maturation of the graafian follicle and production of estradiol.

O   **What limits the secretion of ACTH and corticotropin-releasing factor (CRF)?**

Circulating levels of ACTH.

O   **What factors can alter the diurnal pattern of secretion of ACTH and serum cortisol?**

Periods of stress, such as acute illness, trauma, fever and hypoglycemia.

O   **GH is released in bursts at what specific times?**

3 to 4 hours after meals and during stage III and IV sleep.

O   **Where do the endogenous opioids, beta-endorphins and met-enkephalins bind?**

To receptors in the brain and spinal cord.

O   **What inhibits the release of prolactin?**

Dopamine.

○ **What is the main physiological stimulus for prolactin release?**

Suckling of the breast.

○ **What drugs interfere with release of dopamine into the pituitary portal circulation and enhance prolactin secretion?**

Metaclopramide, haloperidol, chlorpromazine and reserpine.

○ **What signs and symptoms, related to enlargement of the gland, are associated with a pituitary neoplasm?**

Visual field defects (bitemporal hemianopsia), abnormal extraocular muscle movements and spontaneous CSF rhinorrhea.

○ **What characteristics of pituitary apoplexy are due to hemorrhage?**

Severe headache, sudden visual loss, meningismus, decreased sensorium, bloody CSF and ocular palsy.

○ **What is included in the differential diagnosis of a sellar or parasellar tumor?**

Pituitary adenoma, craniopharyngioma, parasellar meningioma, sarcoidosis, metastatic lesions and gliomas.

○ **In evaluation of a patient with an ACTH deficiency, what test will distinguish a hypothalamic CRH deficiency from a pituitary ACTH deficiency?**

The CRH stimulation test.

○ **What is the diagnosis if there is absence of ACTH responsiveness to CRH?**

A pituitary corticotropin deficiency.

○ *What is the ACTH stimulation test used to evaluate?*

The capacity of the adrenal glands to secrete cortisol.

○ **What tests are used to determine gonadotropin deficiency?**

Simultaneous measurements of FSH, LH and gonadal steroids.

○ **What two tests will stimulate the entire HPA?**

The insulin-induced hypoglycemia test and the glucagon test.

○ **What is suggested by a low circulating gonadal steroid level associated with an inappropriately low gonadotropin level?**

A hypothalamic or pituitary disturbance.

○ *What condition is defined by a relative or absolute insufficiency of vasopressin secretion from the posterior pituitary?*

Diabetes insipidus (DI).

○ **How is the diagnosis of central DI confirmed?**

By the water deprivation test.

O   *What is the treatment of choice for central DI?*

Administration of exogenous vasopressin.

O   **T/F: Vasopressin aids in the treatment of renal DI.**
False.

O   **What are the clinical characteristics of Sheehan's syndrome?**

Postpartum failure to lactate, postpartum amenorrhea and progressive signs and symptoms of adrenal insufficiency and hypothyroidism.

O   **What are the most common types of pituitary adenomas?**

Prolactin-secreting and null-cell (chromophobe adenoma).

O   *What is the most common functional pituitary tumor?*

Prolactinoma.

O   **T/F: Prolactinomas occur more frequently in women.**

True.

O   **What is the most common presenting symptom of prolactinomas in females?**

Secondary amenorrhea.

O   **What percentage of patients with a prolactinoma and secondary amenorrhea have an associated galactorrhea?**

50%.

O   **What is the primary symptom of prolactin secreting tumors in males?**

A decrease in libido.

O   **How is the diagnosis of a prolactin secreting tumor confirmed?**

Radiographic evidence of a pituitary lesion with an elevation of serum prolactin.

O   *What pharmaceutical agent is effective in reducing serum prolactin, reducing tumor mass and inhibiting tumor growth?*

Bromocriptine (a dopaminergic agonist).

O   *What is the etiology of Cushing's disease?*

Hypersecretion of ACTH by the pituitary.

O   **What is the most likely diagnosis in a patient with Cushing's syndrome and a low plasma ACTH level?**

An adrenal tumor.

○ **What does an abnormal high-dose glutamine suppression test suggest?**

An autonomous adrenal adenoma.

○ **T/F: Most patients with Cushing's disease harbor microadenomas that lend themselves to complete surgical resection.**

True.

○ **What is the most common cause of excess GH secretion?**

A GH-secreting pituitary adenoma.

○ **What metabolic manifestations are associated with acromegaly?**

Hypertension, diabetes mellitus, goiter and hyperhidrosis.

○ **What is the basal fasting GH level in a patient with acromegaly?**

Less than 10 ng/ml.

○ **What test confirms the diagnosis of acromegaly?**

The glucose suppression test. (An oral administration of 100 gm of glucose fails to suppress the GH level to less than 5 ng/ml at 60 minutes.)

○ **What is the treatment of choice for patients with a GH-producing pituitary adenoma?**

Surgical excision.

○ **What is the appropriate treatment for a patient with a GH-producing pituitary adenoma who cannot withstand the surgical procedure?**

Long-term treatment with octreotide.

○ **What are the most important hormones to evaluate, prior to surgical excision of a pituitary adenoma, to avoid potential perioperative catastrophe?**

Cortisol and thyroid levels.

○ **What is the best surgical approach to the pituitary?**

The transnasal, transsphenoidal approach.

○ **What is the most common cause of surgical death with the transnasal, transsphenoidal approach?**

Direct injury to the hypothalamus, with delayed mortality attributed to CSF leaks and their attendant septic complications or secondary to vascular injury.

○ **What are the contraindications to the transsphenoidal approach?**

Extensive lateral tumor herniating into the middle fossa with minimal midline mass, ectatic carotid arteries projecting toward the midline and acute sinusitis.

○ **What is the standard dosing regimen of glucocorticoids given to all patients undergoing surgical excision of a pituitary tumor?**

40 mg of intravenous methylprednisolone (or 10 mg dexamethasone) every 6 hours, usually starting the day prior to surgery and continuing for 1 or 2 days postoperatively, followed by a tapering dose regimen.

○   **A 55 year old female is in the ICU one day after pituitary tumor resection when she suddenly develops loss of vision. What is the treatment of choice?**

Emergent transsphenoidal re-exploration.

○   **What is the treatment of choice for a patient with a pituitary tumor who is a poor surgical candidate?**

4000 cGy radiation therapy.

○   **What is the recurrence rate of pituitary tumors treated with radiation therapy?**

50%.

○   **A 51 year old male presents with asymmetric visual field defects, optic atrophy, facial sensory deficits and has a tumor attached to the dura mater. What is the most likely diagnosis?**

Meningioma.

○   *A 45 year old male is in the ICU after sustaining blunt head trauma. He suddenly begins to produce an excessive volume of urine, is markedly thirsty and has an increase in his plasma osmolality. What is the most likely diagnosis?*

DI.

○   **What hormones are synthesized and secreted by the adrenal cortex?**

Cortisol, aldosterone, adrenal androgens and estrogen.

○   **What hormones are synthesized and secreted by the adrenal medulla?**

Epinephrine, norepinephrine, enkephalins, neuropeptide Y and corticotropin-releasing hormone.

○   **What is the pathophysiology of Cushing's syndrome?**

Adrenal corticosteroid hypersecretion.

○   **What is the most likely diagnosis of a patient who presents with palpitations, headaches, emesis, a pounding pulse and retinitis?**

Pheochromocytoma.

○   **What is the embryologic origin of the adrenal cortex?**

Coelomic mesothelial cells.

○   **What is the embryologic origin of the adrenal medulla?**

Ectodermal neural crest cells.

○   **What is the primary neurotransmitter of sympathetic postganglionic fibers?**

Norepinephrine.

○ **What are the glands of Zuckerland?**

Ectopic adrenal medullary cells located lateral to the aorta, near the origin of the inferior mesenteric artery.

○ **What is the arterial supply to the adrenal glands?**

The superior suprarenal artery, inferior suprarenal artery and a branch from the inferior phrenic artery.

○ **What is the innervation of the adrenal medulla?**

Preganglionic sympathetic neurons from the celiac and renal plexuses via splanchnic nerves.

○ **What is the drainage of the right adrenal vein?**

The posterior inferior vena cava.

○ **What is the major site of cortisol metabolism?**

The liver.

○ **Most circulating plasma cortisol is bound to what protein?**

Cortisol binding globulin (CBG), though small amounts are bound to albumin and other plasma proteins.

○ **What conditions cause low levels of plasma CBG?**

Liver disease, multiple myeloma, obesity and the nephrotic syndrome.

○ **What is the effect of glucocorticoids on insulin and glucagon?**

It stimulates production of glucagon and inhibits secretion of insulin.

○ ***What are the physiologic actions of aldosterone?***

Reabsorption of sodium and excretion of potassium, hydrogen and ammonia from the renal tubules. It also stimulates active sodium and potassium transport in epithelial tissues (i.e., sweat glands, gastrointestinal mucosa and salivary glands).

○ ***What is the most common cause of Cushing's syndrome?***

A pituitary microadenoma.

○ ***What tumor most commonly causes ectopic ACTH secretion?***

Small cell carcinoma of the lung.

○ **What is the most common tumor of the pituitary gland?**

A chromophobe adenoma.

○ ***What is the expected result of the dexamethasone suppression test in a patient with an ectopic source of ACTH secretion?***

Dexamthasone should fail to suppress cortisol secretion.

○ **Where are the sex steroids produced?**

In the zona reticulosis of the adrenal cortex.

○   **What is the initial evaluation of a patient suspected of having Cushing's syndrome?**

A urinary free cortisol level (markedly elevated) and a low-dose dexamethasone suppression test (no suppression of cortisol).

○   **What is the most likely diagnosis of a patient with elevated free cortisol levels, an elevated plasma ACTH and persistent elevation of free cortisol after low-dose and high-dose dexamethasone administration?**

An ectopic source of ACTH.

○   **What tests are useful in differentiating hypercortisolism due to pituitary sources of ACTH from those due to ectopic sources of ACTH?**

The dexamethasone suppression test and the metyrapone test.

○   **What is the most common cause of primary hyperaldosteronism?**

A solitary adrenal adenoma.

○   **What enzymatic deficiency is associated with most cases of the adrenogenital syndrome (congenital adrenal hyperplasia)?**

21-hydroxylase.

○   **What is the rate-limiting step in catecholamine synthesis?**

Hydroxylation of tyrosine to dihydroxy-phenylalanine (DOPA) by tyrosine hydroxylase.

○   **What are the characteristics of Nelson's syndrome?**

Marked hyperpigmentation of the skin and visual disturbances.

○   **What is the only chemotherapeutic agent that has been proven to be of some value in the treatment of adrenal carcinoma?**

Mitotane.

○   *What is the most common cause of acute adrenocortical insufficiency?*

Withdrawal of chronic steroid therapy.

○   **What is the most common cause of spontaneous adrenal insufficiency?**

Autoimmune destruction of the adrenal glands (greater than 80%).

○   **What is the most commonly associated disorder in patients with autoimmune adrenocortical insufficiency?**

Hashimoto's thyroiditis.

○   **What is Waterhouse-Freiderichsen syndrome?**

Acute adrenal hemorrhage secondary to sepsis (classically meningococcal).

○ **What is the treatment for a patient suspected of having an adrenal crisis?**

A water-soluble corticosteroid.

○ **What is the most useful test to evaluate a patient suspected of having adrenocortical insufficiency?**

The rapid ACTH stimulation test.

○ **What is the treatment for patients with acute adrenocortical insufficiency?**

Intravenous hydrocortisone (100 mg every 6 hours for 24 hours), correction of volume depletion, dehydration, hypotension, hypoglycemia and correction of precipitating factors.

○ **What is the test of choice to distinguish hyperplasia from an adenoma as the cause of primary hyperaldosteronism?**

Measurement of plasma aldosterone concentration after change in posture. Only patients with an adenoma experience a postural decrease in aldosterone.

○ *What are the classic clinical manifestations of primary hyperaldosteronism?*

Hypertension with spontaneous hypokalemia.

○ **What is the most accurate test for localizing an aldosteronoma?**

Selective catheterization of the adrenal veins with sampling for aldosterone levels.

○ **What is the treatment of choice for patients with an adrenaloma?**

Adrenalectomy.

○ **What is the treatment of choice for patients with idiopathic hyperaldosteronism?**

Medical management with spironolactone, a competitive antagonist of aldosterone (200 to 400 mg/day in divided doses).

○ **What are the major enzymes that metabolize catecholamines?**

Monoamineoxidase (MAO) and catechol-o-methyl transferase (COMT).

○ **What is the treatment of choice for idiopathic hyperaldosteronism refractory to medical management?**

Total or subtotal adrenalectomy.

○ **What is the effect of C-21 deficiency in females? In males?**

It causes pseudohermaphrodites in females and macrogenitosomia praecox (enlarged external genitalia) in males.

○ **What test rules out the diagnosis of congenital adrenal hyperplasia (CAH)?**

Failure of the dexamethasone suppression test.

○ **What stimuli cause adrenal secretion of catecholamines?**

Hypoxemia, hypoglycemia, changes in temperature, pain, shock, CNS injury, local wound factors, endotoxin and severe respiratory acidosis.

❍   **T/F: Malignant pheochromocytomas are more common in men.**

False. They are 3 times more common in females.

❍   **What is the diagnostic test of choice to confirm the clinical suspicion of a pheochromocytoma?**

Urine metanephrines.

❍   **Under what conditions should a patient who is undergoing resection of a pheochromocytoma be given preoperative alpha-blockers?**

If the systemic blood pressure is greater than 200/130, if they have frequent and severe uncontrolled hypertensive attacks or if there is a pronounced decrease in plasma volume.

❍   **What is the incidence of neuroblastoma in children?**

Neuroblastoma represents 7% of all childhood cancers. It is the third most common malignancy in childhood (behind brain tumors and hematopoetic-reticular endothelial cell malignancies).

❍   **What is the most common location of a neuroblastoma?**

Intraabdominal or retroperitoneal (60 to 70%).

❍   **What is a Stage III neuroblastoma?**

One that extends in continuity beyond the midline with bilateral lymph node involvement.

❍   **Complete cures with surgical resection can be obtained for neuroblastomas of what stage(s)?**

Stage I, II and IV-S.

❍   **What is the treatment of choice for a Stage III neuroblastoma?**

Radiation and chemotherapy followed by delayed resection.

❍   **What are the classic electrolyte findings of hyperaldosteronism?**

Hypernatremia and hypokalemia.

❍   **What syndromes are associated with pheochromocytomas?**

MEN-IIa, MEN-IIb, von Recklinghausen's disease, tuberous sclerosis and Sturge-Weber disease.

❍   ***What hormones are secreted by the posterior pituitary?***

Oxytocin and vasopressin.

❍   **What is the action of oxytocin?**

It stimulates uterine contraction during labor and elicits milk ejection by myoepithelial cells of the mammary ducts.

THYROID AND PARATHYROID PEARLS

Little minds are interested in the extraordinary,
great minds in the commonplace.
Elbert Hubbard

○   **What is the most common thyroid abnormality in hospitalized patients with non-thyroidal illness?**

Low T3 concentrations.

○   **What are the most common thyroid abnormalities in patients with severe life-threatening non-thyroidal illness?**

Low T4 and low TSH.

○   **What percentage of T3 is derived from conversion of T4?**

80%.

○   **What is the major thyroid hormone-binding protein?**

Thyronine binding globulin (TBG).

○   **What percentage of T4 and T3 are bound?**

Greater than 99.5%.

○   **What are the components of the widespread changes that can occur in thyroid hormone status during critical illness?**

Alternations in the peripheral metabolism of thyroid hormone, TSH regulation and binding of thyroid hormones to TBG.

○   **What is the major cause of a decreased T3 concentration in patients with a critical illness?**

Impaired peripheral conversion of T4 to T3 secondary to inhibition of the deiodination process.

○   **What single test of thyroid function would substantiate the diagnosis of euthyroid in critically ill patients?**

Reverse T3 (rT3).

○   **What factors decrease TSH secretion?**

Acute and chronic illness, adrenergic agonists, calorie restriction, dopamine and dopamine agonists, surgical stress and thyroid hormone metabolites. Minor decreases occur with carbamazapine, clofibrate, opiates, phenytoin and somatostatin.

○   *A patient with a history of radiation exposure as a child was found to have an enlarged lymph node on physical exam. The lymph node is removed and there is normal appearing thyroid tissue in the lymph node. What is the diagnosis?*

Papillary thyroid cancer.

○   **What is the embryologic origin of the thyroid gland?**

From median downgrowth of the first and second pharyngeal pouches in the area of the foramen cecum.

○   **What is the embryologic origin of the parafollicular cells?**

From the ultimobranchial bodies of the fourth and fifth branchial pouches.

○   **What is the effect of pressor doses of dopamine on TSH regulation?**

It decreases TSH levels to normal in patients with pre-existing hypothyroidism.

○   **What factors increase T4 binding to TBG?**

Systemic factors such as liver disease, porphyria, HIV infection and the following drugs: estrogens, methadone, clofibrate, heroin and tamoxifen.

○   **What factors decrease T4 binding to TBG?**

Glucocorticoids, androgens, salicylates, phenytoin, tegretol and furosemide.

○   **What accounts for the low T4 state seen in critically ill patients?**

A decrease in the binding of T4 to serum protein carriers, decreased TSH level, decreased production of T4 and an increase in the nondeiodinative pathways of T4 metabolism.

○   **What is the value of TSH measurements for the evaluation of thyroid disease in critically ill patients?**

A normal test has a high predictive value for normal thyroid function but an abnormal value of TSH alone is not useful.

○   **What is the free T4 index (FTI)?**

FTI = Total T4 x T3 resin uptake.

○   *What genetic mutation is associated with medullary thyroid cancer?*

Ret Proto Oncogene.

○   *What is the first test after H+P to evaluate a thyroid nodule?*

FNA.

○   **Can radioactive iodine be given safely in pregnancy?**

No.

○   **T/F: FTI is increased in hyperparathyroidism.**

True.

❍ **What does the T3 resin uptake test measure?**

It quantitates the degree of saturation of the binding sites of TBG in the serum by T4 and T3.

❍ **What signs and symptoms are associated with hypothyroidism?**

Decreased mental acuity, hoarseness, somnolence, cold intolerance, dry skin, brittle hair, weight gain, hypothermia, generalized edema, hypoventilation, sinus bradycardia and, possibly, hypertension.

❍ **T/F: Cardiac output (CO) is decreased in hypothyroidism.**

True.

❍ **What are the causes of alveolar hypoventilation in myxedematous hypothyroid patients?**

Respiratory center depression with decreased CO_2 sensitivity, defective respiratory muscle strength and possible airway obstruction due to tongue enlargement.

❍ **What laboratory abnormalities are associated with hypothyroidism?**

Hyponatremia, hypoglycemia, hypercholsterolemia and a normochromic normocytic anemia.

❍ **What hormone should uniformly be given with thyroid replacement in the hypothyroid myxedematous patient?**

Hydrocortisone.

❍ *What are the hemodynamics of thyroid storm?*

Tachycardia, increased CO and decreased systemic vascular resistance (SVR).

❍ *What muscle of the larynx is not innervated by the recurrent laryngeal nerve?*

Cricothyroid- innervated by superior laryngeal nerve.

❍ **All the parathyroids typically receive their blood supply from what artery?**

Inferior thyroid.

❍ **Hyperparathyroidism is associated with which oncogene?**

Prad Oncogene.

❍ **What bone finding is pathognomonic finding for hyperparathyroidism?**

Osteitis fibrosa cystica.

❍ **T/F: Hyperparathyroid is most commonly associated with 4 gland hyperplasia.**

False. Solitary parathyroid adenoma is the most common etiology.

❍ **What are the ophthalmologic signs of hyperthyroidism?**

Exophthalmos, lid lag, lid retraction and periorbital swelling.

❍ **What laboratory findings are associated with hyperthyroidism?**

Hypercalcemia, hypokalemia, hyperglycemia, hypocholesterolemia, microcytic anemia, lymphocytosis, granulocytopenia, hyperbilirubinemia and increased alkaline phosphatase.

O   *What is the initial treatment of thyroid storm?*

Intravenous fluids, hypothermia, acetaminophen, propanolol, propylthiouracil (PTU) and iodine.

O   **What are the CNS manifestations of myxedema?**

Depression, memory loss, ataxia, frank psychosis, myxedema and coma.

O   **What is the mechanism of hyponatremia in hypothyroidism?**

Impaired water excretion related to decreased delivery of sodium and volume to the distal renal tubules secondary to decreased renal blood flow.

O   **What are the common causes of hypothyroidism?**

Cessation of thyroid medication, autoimmune thyroid disease, decreased TSH, radioactive and surgical ablation and iodine deficiency/excess.

O   **What is the first thyroid function test abnormality seen in patients with hypothyroidism?**

TSH elevation (usually associated with a low T4).

O   **What single test would allow for the differentiation of thryotoxicosis from acute destructive viral thryoiditis?**

A radioactive iodine uptake (RAIU) test.

O   **Why is the pulse pressure wide in patients with thyrotoxicosis?**

Increased blood flow and vasodilatation.

O   **What inhibits the release of TSH?**

Elevated circulating levels of T3, T4 and somatostatin.

O   **A 45 year old female presents with a 2 year history of diffuse, tender thyroid enlargement, lethargy and a 20-pound weight gain. What is the most likely diagnosis?**

Hashimoto's thyroiditis.

O   **What is the appropriate treatment for the above patient?**

Thyroid replacement therapy.

O   **How is TSH deficiency diagnosed?**

Simultaneous measurement of basal serum TSH and thyroid.

O   **What test is used to distinguish a hypothalamic defect from a pituitary defect in a patient with hypothyroidism?**

The TRH stimulation test.

O   *What is the appropriate treatment for patients with thyroglossal duct cysts?*

Excision of the entire cyst, as well as the thyroglossal tract to its origin, at the foramen cecum, including the central portion of the hyoid bone.

⭘   **What is the venous drainage of the thyroid gland?**

The superior and middle thyroid veins drain into the internal jugular vein and the inferior thyroid veins drain into the innominate vein.

⭘   *What is the result of unilateral injury to the recurrent laryngeal nerve?*

Hoarseness.

⭘   **What is the most common location of the recurrent laryngeal nerve?**

In the tracheoesophageal groove.

⭘   **What is the result of bilateral injury to the superior laryngeal nerve?**

Swallowing disorders.

⭘   *What is the mechanism of action of propylthiouracil (PTU)?*

PTU interferes with the incorporation of iodine into the tyrosine residues of thyroglobulin, preventing oxidation of iodide to iodine. It also inhibits the peripheral conversion of T4 to T3 and is contraindicated in pregnancy.

⭘   **What percentage of T3 is bound to albumin?**

10%.

⭘   *What is the definitive, non-surgical treatment for Grave's disease?*

131-I radioablation.

⭘   **What are the indications for surgical treatment of Grave's disease?**

Extremely large glands, presence of nodules, women of childbearing age and patients who are opposed to radioiodine.

⭘   **What is the preferred treatment for patients with toxic multinodular goiter?**

Thyroid resection (lobectomy to total thyroidectomy) because 131I treatment often requires repeated doses, does not reduce goiter size and may even cause acute enlargement.

⭘   **A 35 year old female presents with a diffuse, slowly growing goiter, weight gain, fatigue and cold intolerance. What is the most likely diagnosis?**

Hashimoto's thyroiditis.

⭘   *What is the single most important test in the diagnostic work-up of a patient with a solitary thyroid nodule?*

Fine needle aspiration (FNA).

⭘   **A 44 year old male presents with a 5 cm thyroid nodule. FNA returns fluid, the nodule disappears and the cytology is benign. What is the next step in management?**

Total thyroid lobectomy with isthmusectomy should be considered because there is an increased chance of malignancy in large cysts.

O   **A 56 year old male with no risk factors presents with a thyroid nodule. The FNA is non-diagnostic. What is the treatment of choice?**

Thyroid lobectomy with isthmusectomy.

O   **What percentage of patients with usual papillary carcinoma (greater than 1 cm) are found to have multicentric disease on pathologic examination of the entire thyroid?**

70 to 80%.

O   **What percentage of patients with papillary carcinoma have cervical lymph node involvement?**

30%.

O   **What factor best correlates with the presence of lymph note metastases in papillary carcinoma?**

Age.

O   **What is the treatment of choice for patients with papillary thyroid cancer without clinical evidence of lymph node metastasis?**

Total thyroidectomy.

O   *A pt is noted to have a very high calcium and a palpable rock hard neck mass, what is your diagnosis?*

Parathyroid adenocarcinoma; Tx: Wide excision with en-block resection of adjacent thyroid tissue.

O   *Classify the MEN syndromes.*

MEN I- PPP- Pancreatic islet cell, Pituitary adenoma, Hyperparathyroidism (4 gland hyperplasia, not adenoma).
MEN IIa- Medullary thyroid, Pheocromocytoma, & Hyperparathyroidism.
MEN IIb- Medullary thyroid, Pheo, Mucosal neuromas/ Marfan Syndrome.

O   **A 36 year old female presents with a 3 cm papillary carcinoma and no clinical evidence of lymph node involvement. She was treated with a total thyroidectomy. What adjuvant therapy is indicated?**

TSH suppression with thyroid hormone, radioiodine ablation with 131I, follow-up scan 6 months after ablation with thyroglobulin levels and physical examination.

O   **Follicular carcinoma metastases occur primarily by what route?**

Hematogenous dissemination to the lungs, bones and other peripheral tissues.

O   **How is the pathologic diagnosis of follicular thyroid carcinoma confirmed?**

Identification of vascular or capsular invasion by the tumor from histologic sections.

O   **What are the indications for adjuvant thyroid hormone in patients with well-differentiated thyroid carcinoma?**

All patients with well-differentiated carcinoma should be treated with thyroid hormone to suppress TSH for life, regardless of the extent of their surgery.

○   **What is the surgical treatment for medullary thyroid carcinoma (MTC)?**

Total thyroidectomy with central node dissection, lateral cervical lymph node sampling of palpable nodes and a modified radical neck dissection, if positive.

○   *A germ-line defect in what gene is responsible for multiple endocrine neoplasias (MEN 2A and MEN 2B) and familiar medullary thyroid carcinoma (FMTC)?*

The RET proto-oncogene.

○   **T/F: Exposure to low-dose radiation therapy is considered a risk factor for thyroid carcinoma.**

True.

○   **What are the histochemical characteristics of MTC?**

Congo red dye positive, apple-green birefringence consistent with amyloid, immunohistochemistry positive for cytokeratins, CEA and calcitonin.

○   *A patient with MTC has a high urinary vanillylmandelic acid (VMA) and an enlarged left adrenal gland. What is the next step in management?*

Medical management with alpha- and beta-blockers, if necessary, followed by resection of the left adrenal gland. This should be performed before the thyroid surgery.

○   *What is the embryological origin of the parathyroid glands?*

The inferior parathyroid glands originate from the third pharyngeal pouch and the superior thyroid glands originate from the fourth pharyngeal pouch.

○   *What is the arterial blood supply to the parathyroids?*

It is usually from the inferior thyroid artery. Occasionally it can arise from the superior thyroid artery, thyroid ima artery or arteries in the larynx, esophagus or mediastinum.

○   *Where are the inferior parathyroids located?*

They are usually more ventral than the superior glands and lie close to or within that portion of the thymus gland that extends from the inferior pole of the thyroid gland into the chest. They are typically located inferior to the junction of the inferior thyroid artery.

○   **What is the effect of PTH on the intestinal absorption of calcium?**

PTH stimulates vitamin D hydroxylation in the kidney.

○   **Where is calcitonin produced?**

In the parafollicular cells (C cells) of the thyroid.

○   **A 48 year old male has a serum calcium of 13 mg/dl and a serum PTH of 400 mEq/ml. What is the most likely diagnosis?**

Primary hyperparathyroidism.

○   *A 35 year old female has a serum calcium of 8.5 mg/dl, a serum PTH of 400 mEq/ml and a serum creatinine of 5.6 mg/dl. What is the most likely diagnosis?*

Secondary hyperparathyroidism.

○   **What are the indications for parathyroid exploration in patients with asymptomatic or minimally symptomatic hyperparathyroidism?**

1.   Age less than 50.
2.   Markedly elevated serum calcium.
3.   History of an episode of life-threatening hypercalcemia.
4.   Decreased creatinine clearance.
5.   Nephrolithiasis.
6.   Markedly elevated 24-hour urinary calcium excretion.
7.   Substantially decreased bone mass.
8.   The patient requests surgery.
9.   Poor follow-up expected.
10. Coexistent illness complicating conservative management.

○   **What percentage of patients with primary hyperparathyroidism have a single adenoma?**

80%.

○   **During exploration for primary hyperparathyroidism, 3 normal parathyroid glands are found but the fourth cannot be identified. What is the next step in management?**

Extend the exploration through the existing excision, to include the central neck between the carotids, posteriorly to the vertebral body, superiorly to the level of the pharynx and carotid bulb and inferiorly into the mediastinum.

○   **What intraoperative modality may assist in locating an intrathyroidal parathyroid gland?**

Ultrasound.

○   **What is the appropriate management if the fourth parathyroid gland cannot be located by intraoperative ultrasound?**

Terminate the operation for localization studies.

○   *What voice problem will a patient have if there is injury to external branch of superior laryngeal nerve?*

Loss of high pitched tone.

○   **What is the most reliable method of differentiating a parathyroid adenoma from parathyroid hyperplasia?**

Visual inspection of all 4 parathyroid glands.

○   *What are the components of the MEN-1 syndrome?*

Parathyroid hyperplasia (90%), islet cell neoplasms (30% to 80%) and pituitary tumors (15% to 50%).

○   **What is the treatment of choice for patients with hyperparathyroidism associated with MEN-1 or MEN-2?**

Subtotal (three and a half gland) parathyroidectomy or total parathyroidectomy with autotransplantation in the forearm.

○   *What is the treatment of choice for patients with parathyroid carcinoma?*

Radical resection of the involved gland, the ipsilateral thyroid lobe and the regional lymph nodes.

❍ **What preoperative studies should be performed prior to re-operation for persistent or recurrent hyperparathyroidism?**

A 24-hour urinary calcium excretion to rule out familiar hypocalciuric, hypercalcemic hyperparathyroidism. Sestamibi is now the localization study of choice.

❍ **A 25 year old pregnant female, in her 2nd trimester, presents with hyperparathyroidism and a serum calcium of 12 mg/dl. What is the treatment of choice?**

Prompt parathyroid exploration.

❍ **What is the surgical treatment of choice for patients with secondary hyperparathyroidism?**

Subtotal (3 and 1/2) parathyroidectomy or total parathyroidectomy with autotransplantation in the forearm.

❍ **What is the first line therapy for patients with marked hypercalcemia and/or severe symptoms?**

Intravenous hydration followed by furosemide.

❍ **What are the indications for calcium supplementation after thyroid or parathyroid surgery?**

Circumoral paresthesias, anxiety, positive Chvostek's or Trousseau's sign, tetany, ECG changes or serum calcium less than 7.1 ml/dl.

❍ **What percentage of individuals with lingual thyroids have no other thyroid tissue?**

70%.

❍ **What is the immediate treatment for patients with acute symptomatic hypocalcemia?**

Intravenous calcium gluconate.

❍ **In a non-acute setting, what is the maximum useful amount of calcium supplementation?**

2 grams of calcium/day.

❍ **What is the appropriate calcium supplementation if the maximum amount of calcium has already been given and the patient is still hypocalcemic?**

Calcitriol or other vitamin D preparations should be added, if necessary.

❍ *What are the phenotypic abnormalities seen in patients with MEN-2B?*

Medullary thyroid carcinoma, pheochromocytoma, mucosal neuromas, ganglioneuromas and a marfanoid habitus.

TRAUMA AND BURN PEARLS

If you are too smart to pay the doctor, you had better be too smart to get ill.
African proverb

○ **What are the absolute indications for invasive airway management?**

Obstruction, apnea, hypoxia and severe neck trauma.

○ **A trauma patient presents with a decreasing level of consciousness and an enlarging right pupil. What is the most likely diagnosis?**

Uncal herniation with oculomotor nerve compression.

○ **Which cranial nerves are evaluated with the corneal reflex test?**

The ophthalmic, trigeminal and facial nerves.

○ **What are the clinical signs of a basilar skull fracture?**

Periorbital and retroauricular ecchymosis, otorrhea, rhinorrhea, hemotympanum and cranial nerve deficits.

○ **Which sensations are spared in anterior cord syndrome?**

Position, vibratory and, possibly, light touch.

○ **How much airway obstruction is required for inspiratory stridor to become clinically evident?**

70%.

○ **What is the most common cause of shock in patients with blunt chest trauma?**

Pelvic or extremity fracture.

○ *What method of airway control is indicated in a patient with severe maxillofacial trauma?*

Cricothyroidotomy.

○ **What nerve should be avoided during pericardiotomy?**

The phrenic nerve.

○ **A 36 year old female trauma victim presents with a rocking-horse type of ventilation. What is the most likely diagnosis?**

A high spinal cord injury with intercostal muscle paralysis.

○ **A pneumothorax is suspected but does not show up on PA or lateral chest x-rays. What is the next step in evaluation?**

Expiratory films.

199

❍   **What is the most likely cause of a new systolic murmur and ECG infarct pattern in a patient with chest trauma?**

A ventricular septal defect.

❍   **When does the CPK-MB fraction peak in a patient with a cardiac contusion?**

18 to 24 hours after injury.

❍   **What plain film x-ray finding is most suggestive of traumatic rupture of the aorta?**

Deviation of the esophagus greater than 2 cm to the right of the spinous process of T4. (This requires nasogastric intubation to be demonstrated.)

❍   **What is the basic disorder contributing to the pathophysiology of compartment syndrome?**

Increased pressure within closed tissue spaces and compromising blood flow to muscles and nerve tissue.

❍   **What are the late signs and symptoms of compartment syndrome?**

The compartment is tense, indurated and erythematous, with slow capillary refill, pallor and pulselessness.

❍   *What signs and symptoms are associated with compartment syndrome involving the superficial posterior compartment of the leg?*

Pain on active and passive foot dorsiflexion and plantar flexion and hypesthesia of the lateral aspect of the foot (sural nerve).

❍   **What bullet characteristics determine the degree of tissue injury?**

Yaw, deformation and fragmentation (of missile and bone).

❍   **What is the proper approach for a diagnostic peritoneal lavage (DPL) in a trauma patient with a fractured pelvis?**

Via a supraumbilical incision.

❍   *In blunt trauma there is suspected diaphragm rupture. What is a quick and easy test?*

Insert NGT and obtain an x-ray. If NGT in chest you have your answer.

❍   *What are the indications for thoracotomy for hemothorax?*

1500 cc out initially (some say 1000), > 200cc/hr x 4 hrs, unstable, incomplete drainage after two functional chest tubes.

❍   **Define the landmarks for the zones of the neck?**

I-below cricoid; II- cricoid to angle of jaw; III above angle of mandible.

❍   *What findings represent a positive DPL in blunt trauma?*

Greater than 100,000 RBCs/mm^3, a WBC count greater than 500 cells/mm^3 or the presence of bile, bacteria or vegetable material.

❍   **What is the diagnostic test of choice for patients with a zone II penetrating neck injury?**

Classically operative exploration, however, with the ready availability of CT scan at most trauma centers, these studies are often done with constrast in stable patients with zone II neck injuries.

O   **What is the initial treatment for patients with acute spinal cord injury?**

30 mg/kg of methylprednisolone over 15 minutes in the first hour, followed by 5.4 mg/kg/hr over the next 23 hours.

O   **What percentage of cervical spine fractures are seen on lateral x-rays of the neck?**

90%.

O   **How much anterior subluxation is normal on an adult lateral cervical spine x-ray?**

Approximately 3.5 mm.

O   **What is a clay-shoveler's fracture?**

An avulsion fracture of the spinous process of C7, C6 or T1.

O   ***What are the characteristics of spinal shock?***

Sudden areflexia that is transient and distal, blood pressure of 80 to 100 mm Hg and paradoxical bradycardia.

O   ***A 22 year old male was involved in a high-speed motor vehicle accident (MVA). The patient has been stabilized and secondary survey reveals blood at the urethral meatus. What is the diagnostic test of choice?***

A retrograde urethrogram.

O   **What are the most commonly injured genitourinary organs?**

The kidneys and bladder.

O   **What mechanisms of injury creates wounds that are most susceptible to infection?**

Compression and tension injuries.

O   **Bacterial endocarditis, secondary to soft tissue infections, is most commonly caused by what organisms?**

Staphylococcus aureus and Staphylococcus epidermidis.

O   **What factors increase the likelihood of wound infection?**

Contamination, stellate or crushing wounds, wounds longer than 5 cm or older than 6 hours and infection prone anatomic sites.

O   **What is the most common Salter-Harris fracture?**

Type II.

O   **What tarsal bone is most commonly fractured?**

The calcaneus.

O   **What percentage of patients with peripheral arterial injuries have palpable distal pulses?**

20%.

○   **Which patellar fractures require orthopedic consultation?**

Displaced transverse fractures, comminuted fractures and open fractures.

○   **What is the most common type of ankle injury?**

Anterior talofibular sprains.

○   **Which pelvic fracture is most likely to result in severe hemorrhage?**

Vertical sheer fractures.

○   **What is the preferred timing of intramedullary fixation in the multiply-injured trauma patient with a femur fracture?**

Within 24 hours.

○   **What is the incidence of compartment syndrome in patients with an open tibial fracture?**

10%.

○   **What associated injuries must be considered in the presence of calcaneal fractures?**

Vertebral compression or burst fractures.

○   **With regard to patients with traumatic hand injuries, what is the most important treatment to prevent infection?**

Adequate debridement.

○   **What is the appropriate method of transport of amputated digits?**

They should be stored on saline moistened gauze, in a plastic bag and placed on ice.

○   **T/F: Pregnant women are at a higher risk for developing disseminated intravascular coagulation (DIC) following trauma than nonpregnant women.**

True.

○   **What impact velocity is required to penetrate bone?**

Approximately 200 ft/sec.

○   **T/F: Nerve injury associated with low velocity missile wounding is usually permanent.**

False.

○   *What factors indicate the need for an angiogram after penetrating trauma to an extremity?*

Absent or diminished pulse, a cold extremity, difference in extremity systolic pressures, the presence of a bruits or thrills and the proximity to major vessels.

○   **What percentage of gunshot related arterial injuries are associated with concomitant nerve injury?**

70%.

O   **A 40 year old male unrestrained driver in a high-speed MVA presents with multiple rib fractures and is in respiratory distress with paradoxical chest motion. What is the treatment of choice?**

Immediate intubation with volume-controlled ventilation.

O   **What is the late amputation rate in patients with an open fracture associated with vascular or neurologic injury?**

75%.

O   **Injury to what structure is most commonly responsible for persistent hemorrhage requiring a thoracotomy?**

An intercostal artery.

O   **What percentage of patients with blunt chest trauma and a flail chest also have a pulmonary contusion?**

Greater than 90%.

O   **T/F: Steroids are indicated in the treatment of pulmonary contusion.**

False.

O   **Where does blunt rupture of the trachea most frequently occur?**

Within 2.5 cm of the carina.

O   **What valvular abnormality is most commonly seen in patients after blunt chest trauma?**

Aortic insufficiency.

O   **What is the most common site of blunt esophageal rupture?**

The distal third.

O   **What is the best surgical approach for patients with proximal thoracic esophageal injuries?**

A right posterolateral thoracotomy.

O   **What is a second degree corrosive esophageal burn?**

A transmucosal burn without muscle involvement.

O   **What is the incidence of associated intrathoracic injuries in patients with a fracture of the scapula or first or second rib?**

Greater than 50%.

O   **A 19 year old female presents with a stab wound to the left fifth intercostal space, hypotension and the water-bottle sign is seen on chest x-ray. What is the most likely diagnosis?**

Pericardial tamponade.

O   ***What are the initial cardiovascular effects of increased intracranial pressure (ICP)?***

Bradycardia and hypertension.

❍   **What are the clinical manifestations of the postpericardiotomy syndrome?**

Fever, chest pain, pericardial effusion and a pericardial rub.

❍   **A 35 year old male is in the ICU following major blunt chest trauma and is being mechanically ventilated. He develops sudden onset of lateralizing neurologic signs. What diagnosis must be considered?**

Air embolism.

❍   **What physical examination finding confirms the diagnosis of air embolism?**

Air bubbles in the retinal vessels.

❍   **A 26 year old trauma patient presents in extremis. Emergency thoracotomy is performed and the patient is found to have air in his coronary vessels. What life-saving maneuver must be attempted?**

Clamping of the hilum of the affected lung.

❍   **T/F: Prolonged external loss of chyle can lead to severe malnutrition, electrolyte loss and T-cell suppression.**

True.

❍   **What is the only absolute contraindication to DPL?**

Obvious need for laparotomy.

❍   **What injuries are most commonly missed by CT scans?**

Injuries to a hollow viscus, the pancreas and the diaphragm.

❍   **What is the most commonly injured organ secondary to penetrating trauma to the abdomen?**

The small bowel.

❍   **When is primary repair of a colon injury not warranted?**

In the presence of gross fecal contamination, shock, massive blood loss, other associated abdominal injuries or delay in diagnosis greater than 8 hours.

❍   **T/F: In the management of patient with colon injuries, the incidence of postoperative intraabdominal sepsis is higher in patients undergoing primary repair versus those undergoing colostomy.**

False.

❍   **T/F: A 21 year old male presents with a stab wound to the abdomen. The secondary survey reveals rectal blood. A negative proctoscopy rules out rectal injury.**

False.

❍   **What are the important factors in the management of patients with penetrating rectal injuries?**

Diversion, drainage and debridement.

❍   **What percentage of patients with pancreatic injuries have associated intraabdominal injuries?**

Greater than 90%.

O **T/F: Serum amylase is a useful marker for ruling out pancreatic injury.**

False.

O *What is the emergency treatment of choice for a patient with a tension pneumothorax?*

Needle decompression at the second intercostal space in the midclavicular line.

O *What is the treatment of choice for a patient with a pancreatic transection distal to the superior mesenteric artery?*

Distal pancreatectomy.

O *What injury is suggested by retroperitoneal gas on plane abdominal radiograph, along the right psoas margin or over the right pole of the kidney?*

A duodenal injury.

O **A 50 year old male presents to the emergency room in extremis with a stab wound to the right chest and pulsatile bleeding. What is the proper surgical approach?**

A left anterolateral thoracotomy.

O **What is the procedure of choice for a patient with a duodenal injury that disrupts the ampulla but spares the pancreatic head?**

Primary reimplantation of the distal bile duct and pancreatic duct into the posterior duodenal wall.

O **Patients with small duodenal lacerations are best treated in what manner?**

A 2-layer transverse primary closure.

O **T/F: An acceptable means of mobilizing the pancreas, in order to inspect the gland for trauma, is to ligate the inferior mesenteric vein.**

True.

O **What is the mechanism of injury in aortic transection?**

Sudden deceleration (i.e., MVA) that leads to the development of shear forces between the mobile aortic arch and the fixed descending aorta.

O **What is the most reliable test to identify patients with cardiac contusion who are at risk for complications?**

ECG.

O **What is the treatment for patients with a pancreatic contusion, without ductal injury?**

Wide drainage.

O **What are the indications for pancreaticoduodenectomy in abdominal trauma?**

Massive hemorrhage from the head of the pancreas or adjacent vascular structures, severe ductal injury in the head of pancreas and combined injuries of the duodenum and head of the pancreas.

O   **What is the procedure of choice for a patient with a pancreatic injury to the right of the superior mesenteric artery (SMA), without injury to the ampulla?**

Oversewing of the proximal pancreas, with a Roux-en-Y pancreaticojejunostomy, to the distal pancreas or ductal ligation with wide drainage.

O   **What is the coiled spring sign?**

The radiographic appearance of a duodenal hematoma on an upper GI contrast study.

O   **T/F: Opening Gerota's fascia, prior to obtaining vascular control, increases the nephrectomy rate.**

False.

O   *What is the initial treatment for a patient with a duodenal hematoma?*

Observation and nasogastric suction.

O   **When is primary closure of the duodenum contraindicated?**

In patients with gunshot injuries of greater than 50% of the duodenal circumference or when an associated bile duct injury is present.

O   **What is the overall mortality rate for patients with grade III liver injuries?**

25%.

O   **Anomalous origins of the common hepatic and right hepatic arteries frequently arise from what artery?**

The superior mesenteric artery.

O   **What is the indication for the Pringle maneuver?**

To demonstrate that hepatic hemorrhage is coming from the hepatic artery or portal vein, as opposed to the hepatic veins or inferior vena cava.

O   **What is the treatment of choice for patients with a complex bile duct injury?**

A roux-en-Y choledochojejunostomy or a hepatojejunostomy.

O   **What is the most appropriate treatment for an unstable patient found to have a liver injury during exploratory laparotomy?**

Perihepatic packing.

O   **What is the most frequent indication for exploratory laparotomy following blunt trauma?**

Splenic injury.

O   **What percentage of splenic injuries in children can be managed expectantly?**

Greater than 90%.

O   **What organisms are most commonly associated with overwhelming postsplenectomy sepsis (OPS)?**

Pneumococcus, meningococcus and Haemophilus influenza.

❍ **What is the mortality rate for overwhelming postsplenectomy sepsis?**

50%.

❍ **How much of the spleen is required to maintain immunologic competence?**

One-third.

❍ **T/F: Mandibular condyle fractures are usually adequately treated with closed reduction.**

True.

❍ **What are the contraindications for the use of laparoscopy for evaluation of the abdomen in a trauma patient?**

Multiple previous operations, shock or head injury with elevated ICP.

❍ **What is the most commonly missed injury with use of laparoscopy for evaluation of the abdomen in trauma patients?**

A hollow viscus injury.

❍ **Which retroperitoneal hematomas require mandatory exploration after blunt abdominal trauma?**

Those centrally located.

❍ **What determines surgical management of retroperitoneal hematomas?**

The zonal distribution and the mechanism of injury.

❍ **What are the most rapid means of assessing intravascular volume status?**

Level of consciousness and pulse.

❍ **What are the soft signs that indicate a possible arterial injury?**

Neurologic deficit, history of hypotension, nonpulsatile hematoma and injury in proximity to a major artery.

❍ **What fractures are most commonly associated with compartment syndrome?**

Closed tibia and supracondylar humerus fractures.

❍ **T/F: Mesenteric hematomas larger than 2 cm require exploration.**

True.

❍ **What is a Jefferson fracture?**

An atlantal burst fracture.

❍ **A 33 year old male presents with hematemesis and jaundice 3 weeks after having sustained a gunshot wound to the liver. What is the most likely diagnosis?**

Hemobilia.

❍ **What injuries are associated with inflation of air bags?**

Corneal abrasions, keratitis, face and neck abrasions and cervical spine fractures.

○   *A patient presents to the emergency department after an MVA with neck hyperextension injury unable to move or feel his upper extremities, yet the lower extremities remain intact. What is the most likely diagnosis?*

Central cord syndrome.

○   **What is the single most important determinant of outcome in patients following pancreatic injury?**

Presence of a pancreatic ductal injury.

○   **What movements of the lower extremity are possible in a patient with transection of the sciatic nerve?**

Flexion and adduction of the thigh.

○   **What serious complication may result from delay in reduction of a dislocated hip?**

Avascular necrosis of the femoral head.

○   **Most burn injuries occur in what age group?**

Children less than 2 years of age.

○   **T/F: Burn injuries occur more commonly in the lower socioeconomic population.**

True.

○   **What is the most common mechanism of burn to children less than 5 years of age?**

Scalding.

○   **What percentage of total body surface area (TBSA) burn requires hospitalization?**

15% second degree burns or 5% third degree.

○   **What factors increase the mortality rate of burned patients?**

Children less than 4 years of age, size of burn, inhalation injury, concomitant injury or disease and prolonged time from burn to admission.

○   **What is the most common cause of early instability in burn patients?**

Severe inhalation injury.

○   **What is the pathophysiologic mechanism by which red blood cells are damaged in burn patients?**

Burn-induced complement activation with subsequent oxygen radical production.

○   **When does capillary permeability return to normal in a burned patient?**

During the second 24 hours post-burn.

○   *What is the best way to determine adequate fluid resuscitation in a burn victim?*

Urine output.

❍   **A 40 year old 70 kg male sustained a 30% TBSA second degree burn. In route to the hospital he received 200 ml crystalloid. What should his fluid rate be upon admission?**

500 ml/hr.

❍   **Which organ has the worst perfusion in burned patients?**

The kidney.

❍   **What should the urine output be for a patient who has suffered an electrical burn and has reddish urine?**

100 to 150 ml/hr.

❍   **What is the best measure of intravascular volume capacity and the ability to infuse additional fluid to a burned patient?**

Pulmonary capillary wedge pressure (PCWP).

❍   **What serious associated injury is the most frequently seen in burn patients?**

Inhalation injury.

❍   **What is the fluid requirement in a burn patient who has also suffered an inhalation injury compared to a patient who has not?**

An inhalation injured burn patient requires 40 to 50% more fluid volume.

❍   *At what point in resuscitation of burn patients should pharmacologic adjuncts be administered?*

If the patient remains oliguric with a PCWP of 18 to 20 mm Hg.

❍   **What is the estimated evaporative water loss in a 75 kg male with a 40% TBSA second degree burn?**

9 liters.

❍   **What is the proper location for escharotomy in patients with circumferential full-thickness extremity burns?**

The mid-medial and mid-lateral lines, down to and just through the subdermal fascial attachments.

❍   **What is the mechanism of increased pulmonary vascular permeability in burn patients?**

Activation of the complement system, resulting in chemotaxis and sequestration of neutrophils within the pulmonary capillaries and subsequent hydroxyl radical formation.

❍   **What histological findings are associated with inhalation injury?**

Edema, progressive tracheobronchitis with pseudomembrane formation and airway obstruction.

❍   **What is the major cause of hypoxia in fire-related deaths in urban areas?**

Carbon monoxide poisoning.

❍   **What is the most accurate diagnostic test for inhalation injury?**

Bronchoscopy.

○   **At what time post-inhalation injury is pulmonary edema at its maximum?**

Within 24 to 48 hours.

○   **What percentage of patients with large airway inhalation injury will have a concomitant parenchymal injury?**

85%.

○   **What are the primary complications of inhalation injury?**

Pneumonia, atalectasis and pulmonary edema.

○   **What are the indications for mechanical ventilatory support in the burn patient with an inhalation injury?**

PaO2 less than 60 mm Hg on an FIO2 of greater than 0.4, PCO2 greater than 50 mm Hg and respiratory distress.

○   **What is the major concern in patients with isolated pelvic injuries?**

The possibility of exsanguination.

○   **What agent is most effective for cleansing and decontaminating burn wounds?**

Chlorhexidine.

○   **What are the most common signs of burn wound infection?**

Dark brown or violaceous discoloration of the wound and hemorrhage into the subeschar tissue.

○   **Peripheral hemorrhagic infarcts of ecthyma gangrenosum are specific for what type of infection?**

Pseudomonas.

○   **What are the most common fungal organisms that cause burn wound sepsis?**

Phycomycetes and aspergillus.

○   **What is the single most important sign of burn wound infection on biopsy?**

The presence of microbial organisms in unburned, viable tissue.

○   **What topical antimicrobial agent does not penetrate eschars?**

Silver nitrate.

○   **What are the major mediators of the hypermetabolic response in burn patients?**

Catecholamines.

○   **T/F: Thermal injuries suppress thyroid hormone.**

True.

❍ **What are the predominant cytokines that promote wound healing and amplify the hypermetabolic response?**

IL-1, IL-6, TNF and IFN-gamma.

❍ **What is the best source of non-protein calories for a burn patient?**

Carbohydrates.

❍ **What is the daily caloric requirement for a 75 kg male with a 20% TBSA burn?**

2,675 Kcal (25 Kcal/kg + 40 Kcal per percent TBSA burn).

❍ **T/F: Wound infection is the most common cause of mortality in burn patients.**

False. Pneumonia is more common.

❍ **What is the incidence of stress ulceration of the stomach or duodenum (Curling's ulcer) in a patient with 35% or greater TBSA burn?**

20%.

❍ **What type of bodily tissue offers the most resistance to current flow?**

Bone.

❍ **What is the hallmark of an electrical injury?**

Extensive deep tissue damage that is far out of proportion to the visible cutaneous burn.

❍ **What are the mechanisms by which hydrofluoric acid produces toxicity?**

Hydrogen ions induce protein coagulation and free fluoride ions cause liquefaction and penetrate deeply to form salts with magnesium and calcium.

❍ **What is the most effective treatment for patients with hydrofluoric acid burns?**

Administration of calcium gluconate to the burn wound.

❍ **What is the treatment of choice for skin that has come into contact with phenol?**

A 50% solution of polyethylene glycol followed by copious water irrigation.

❍ **Why are alkaline burns usually more invasive than acid burns?**

Alkaline burns cause damage by liquefaction necrosis. Thus, a barrier of coagulated protein does not form.

❍ **What type of tar contains the greatest amount of volatile substances and causes the most marked tissue damage?**

Coal tar.

❍ **What is the best position for a burned body part to prevent contracture?**

The anti-deformity posture.

❍ **What is the effect of prophylactic antibiotics on burn wound sepsis?**

They promote selection of antibiotic-resistant bacteria.

O   **How is the diagnosis of burn wound sepsis confirmed?**

Presence of greater than 100,000 organism/gram of tissue.

O   **What percentage of burns in children admitted to hospitals are purposefully inflicted?**

10%.

O   **What is the immediate treatment for patients with chemical burns?**

Irrigation with large amounts of water.

ORTHOPEDIC AND HAND SURGERY PEARLS

Caution: Cape does not enable user to fly.
Batman costume warning label

○ **During normal walking, both feet are touching the ground in what phase of the gait cycle?**

The swing phase.

○ *What severe complication is associated with cast treatment of unstable supracondylar humerus fractures in children?*

Volkmann's ischemic contracture of the forearm.

○ **What serum proteins influence bone induction?**

Platelet-derived growth factor, transforming growth factor-beta, osteogenin and fibroblast growth factor.

○ **What orthopedic procedure is associated with the greatest improvement in quality of life?**

Total hip arthroplasty.

○ **What autosomal dominant syndrome is characterized by aplasia of the clavicles, increased transverse cranial diameter and delayed closure of the fontanelles?**

Cleidocranial dysostosis.

○ **What are the most sensitive tests to evaluate the integrity of the anterior cruciate ligament?**

The Lachman test and the anterior drawer test.

○ **What is the etiology of ganglion cysts?**

Protrusion of a joint capsule or tendon sheath that fills with a jelly-like fluid.

○ **What is the most common location of ganglion cysts?**

At the scapholunate interosseous ligament.

○ *Injury to the ulnar nerve near the elbow has what effect on hand function?*

Weakness of adduction and abduction of digits 2 through 5.

○ **What is the appropriate treatment for a 2 year old boy who walks awkwardly because his feet point inward?**

Conservative therapy and counseling.

○   **What is the etiology of trigger fingers?**

Tenosynovitis in the region of the MCP joint.

○   **What is the most common location of a clavicular fracture?**

At the junction of the middle and distal thirds of the clavicle.

○   **What is the most common presentation of an acute anterior cruciate ligament tear?**

Pain and acute hemarthrosis.

○   **What is the first material formed by osteoblasts at the fracture site?**

Woven bone.

○   **What is the result of untreated joint tuberculosis?**

Joint destruction, deformity and pain.

○   *Dislocations risk nerve injury. What nerves must be tested in hip and shoulder dislocations?*

Hip- Sciatic.
Shoulder- axillary. Sensation on top of shoulder.

○   *Humeral neck fracture is associated with what nerve injury?*

Radial. May present with weak wrist extension.

○   **What is the most frequently isolated organism from hand infections?**

Staphylococci.

○   *What nerve is most commonly injured with anterior glenohumeral dislocation?*

The axillary nerve.

○   **The biceps brachii muscle receives its major innervation from what spinal segment?**

C5.

○   **When do most patients with fat embolism syndrome develop clinical signs?**

Within 48 hours of injury.

○   **What is the proper treatment for an athlete with isolated medial collateral ligament disruption?**

Immobilization in 45°of flexion for 2 to 3 weeks followed by bracing and progressive increase in range-of-motion.

○   **What is a boutonniere deformity of the finger?**

Proximal interphalangeal (PIP) flexion and distal interphalangeal (DIP) hyperextension.

○   **What is the underlying cause of osteopetrosis?**

Decreased osteoclast activity.

❍ *What is the most important finding in establishing the diagnosis of fat embolism syndrome?*

A low PaO2 after long bone fracture.

❍ **What is the rate of axonal nerve growth following injury?**

About 1 mm/day.

❍ **When is ORIF indicated for closed humeral shaft fractures?**

If there is marked displacement or interposition of soft tissue.

❍ **What joint is involved in a Bennett's fracture?**

The carpometacarpal (CMC) joint of the thumb.

❍ **What is the most effective method for diagnosis and treatment of knee ligament injuries?**

Arthroscopy.

❍ **What are the long-term effects of rheumatoid arthritis (RA) on the hand?**

Ulnar deviation and subluxation of the metacarpal-phalangeal joints, rupture of tendons and contracture of intrinsic muscles.

❍ *What are the indications for immediate surgical intervention in a patient with complete dislocation of the knee?*

Popliteal artery injury, open dislocation or irreducible dislocation.

❍ **What is the appropriate treatment for a child with a supracondylar elbow fracture?**

Manipulation, closed reduction and immobilization of the arm at 90° with slight pronation.

❍ **T/F: Trabecular bone remodeling occurs much more rapidly than cortical bone remodeling.**

True.

❍ **What is the appropriate management of a lower extremity sarcoma less than 10 cm in size?**

Limb-sparing resection and radiation therapy.

❍ **What is the most common cause of posterior dislocations of the shoulder?**

Epileptiform seizures or electroshock therapy.

❍ **What is the appropriate management of gonococcal arthritis?**

A 2-week course of penicillin and joint immobilization.

❍ *What type of collagen is found in cartilage?*

Type II.

❍ **What percentage of patients with fractures of the neck of the talus will develop avascular necrosis?**

At least 50%.

○   *What are the characteristics of Paget's disease of bone?*

Increased bone formation and resorption. The new bone becomes enlarged with thickened cortices and trabeculae yet is mechanically weak.

○   **What is the most common primary bone malignancy?**

Osteosarcoma.

○   **What is the appropriate antibiotic prophylaxis for a farming-related open tibia fracture?**

Triple-antibiotic therapy and tetanus prophylaxis.

○   **What is the etiology of Dupuytren's contractures?**

Proliferation of the palmar fascia.

○   **What is the appropriate treatment if ischemia is suspected in a casted patient?**

Cutting a window into the cast.

○   **Which digits are most commonly affected by Dupuytren's contractures?**

The ring and small fingers.

○   **What vertebrae are most commonly affected by cervical disc disease?**

C4, C5 and C6.

○   **What is the principle form of fracture healing?**

Membranous ossification.

○   **What factors affect bone remodeling in fractures in the pediatric age group?**

The age of the child, the distance of the fracture from the physis and the plane of the deformity in relation to the plane of motion of the nearest joint.

○   **What are the late findings of RA?**

Subluxation of the involved joints and joint deformity.

○   *Fracture of the distal radius is associated with injury to what nerve?*

The median nerve.

○   **What is the treatment of choice for cervical disc disease?**

Cervical traction, NSAIDs and a cervical collar.

○   **What is the appropriate treatment for cervical disc disease following failed medical management?**

Cervical discectomy and spine fusion.

○   **What are the classic symptoms of carpal tunnel syndrome?**

Pain, numbness and tingling in the median nerve distribution, weakness of the thenar muscles and worsening of symptoms at night.

❍ **What is the function of the osteoblast and the osteoclast?**

Osteoblast- Build bone.
Osteoclast- Break down bone.

❍ **L4-L5 disc will give which nerve root compression?**

L5 (a level below).

❍ **The following root compressions give what symptoms?**

L4- weak knee jerk; L5- weak toes dorsiflexion; S1- weak toe plantar flexion, weak ankle jerk.

❍ *What is the etiology of Volkmann's ischemic contracture?*

Injury or constriction of the brachial artery, usually from injuries about the elbow.

❍ *What is the maximum intraoperative tourniquet time in hand surgery?*

2 hours.

❍ **What are the late complications of Volkmann's ischemic contracture?**

Obliteration of the radial pulse and anoxia of the median and ulnar nerves.

❍ **Following carpal tunnel release, how should the wrist be immobilized?**

With the wrist in 30° of extension, the MP joints in 70° of flexion and the IP joints in extension or minimal flexion.

❍ **What are the characteristics of a Montaggia's fracture?**

Fracture of the proximal ulna with subluxation of the radial head.

❍ **Single digits are usually only replanted in what patients?**

Children.

❍ **What are the radiographic findings associated with osteoarthritis?**

Joint-space narrowing, subchondral sclerosis, osteophytes and cyst formation. Joint deformity and malalignment may also occur.

❍ *What is the current standard of care for patients with an osteosarcoma?*

Een bloc resection with neo-adjuvant or adjuvant therapy.

❍ **What muscles comprise the rotator cuff?**

The teres minor, infraspinatus, supraspinatus and subscapularis.

❍ **What is the innervation of the flexor digitorum profundus to the ring and little fingers?**

The ulnar nerve.

❍   **What are the advantages of internal stabilization of an open fracture?**

It minimizes soft tissue trauma, provides a stable environment for soft-tissue healing, provides pain relief and increases the likelihood of fracture healing.

❍   *What is the most effective therapy for full thickness burns of the hands?*

Early excision and skin grafting.

❍   **What type of pediatric fracture involves partial disruption of the cortex and usually heals with conservative management?**

Greenstick fractures.

❍   **Absence of the knee jerk is suggestive of what process?**

Compression at the L3-L4 level.

❍   **What type of scoliosis most often results in paraplegia?**

Untreated congenital scoliosis.

❍   **What is the diagnostic test of choice for meniscus tears?**

MRI.

❍   **What are the most important prognostic factors in idiopathic scoliosis?**

The age of onset and the site of the curve.

❍   **What are the hallmarks of chondromalacia?**

Softening and discoloration of the patellar cartilage.

❍   **What is the most common cause of pyogenic osteomyelitis of the vertebral column?**

Hematogenous spread of Staphylococcus aureus.

❍   **What maximal period of anoxia is still compatible with successful replantation of the upper extremity?**

Up to 20 hours.

❍   **What is the most common cause of spondylolisthesis?**

A structural defect in the pars interarticularis (spondylolysis).

❍   **What percentage of patients with posterior hip dislocations will develop avascular necrosis of the femoral head?**

20%.

❍   *Posterior dislocation of the knee and an abnormal distal puls exam mandates what study be ordered?*

Arteriogram.

○ **What fractures are likely to cause compartment syndrome?**

Tibia fx, supracondylar humerus fx, calcaneous fx.

○ **What is Volkmann's contracture?**

Compartment syndrome of deep forearm flexor secondary to supracondylar humerus fracture.

○ *Which artery and which nerve may be compromised in Volkmann's contracture?*

Median nerve, and Anterior interosseous artery.

○ **What is the most important factor related to development of avascular necrosis of the femoral head following posterior hip dislocations?**

Delay in reduction.

○ **What is the appropriate treatment for radial neck fractures with more than 45° of angulation?**

Open reduction.

○ **What are the disadvantages of internal stabilization of an open fracture?**

Foreign body reaction and infection.

○ **What are the most common locations of stress fractures?**

The femoral neck, the distal second and third metatarsal shafts, the proximal tibia, distal fibula and the calcaneus.

○ **What are the indications for surgical intervention in patients with gout?**

Large, symptomatic, tophaceous deposits and severely involved joints.

○ **What area of the hand and fingers constitutes Zone 2 (no man's land)?**

The area between the MCP joint and the superficialis insertion.

○ **What is the primary constituent of adult cortices?**

Secondary osteonal bone.

○ *Calf pain similar to claudication that does not resolve with rest is suggestive of what entity?*

Spinal stenosis.

○ **What are the indications for prophylactic stabilization of a malignant lesion in the proximal femur?**

Pain refractory to conservative management, lesion diameter greater than 2.5 cm, involvement of 50% of the cortical thickness and avulsion of the lesser trochanter.

○ **What are the nonoperative measures for treatment of Dupuytren's contractures?**

Exercise, local injections of steroids and radiotherapy.

○ **What are the typical clinical manifestations of acromioclavicular injuries?**

Local swelling and tenderness over the joint and a palpable deformity.

○ **What is a gamekeeper's thumb?**

Rupture of the ulnar collateral ligament of the MP joint with resultant instability of the joint to radial-directed force.

○ *What is the treatment of choice for Ewing's sarcoma?*

Chemotherapy plus radiation therapy.

○ **What is the most common site of proximal humeral fractures?**

The surgical neck.

○ **T/F: Fractures of the distal phalanx account for more than one-half of all hand fractures.**

True.

○ **What complications may occur if nerve repair is delayed beyond 2 weeks?**

Retraction of the nerve ends, resulting in the need for nerve grafting.

○ **When is treatment of congenital club foot most successful?**

When performed in infancy.

○ **What is the treatment of choice for club foot in skeletally mature patients?**

Triple arthrodesis.

○ **What is the rationale for internal fixation of a displaced intra-articular fracture?**

Increased joint contact and lower pressure on the cartilage results in a decrease in post-traumatic osteoarthritis, early joint motion and prevention of joint stiffness.

○ **What is a Mallet finger?**

Injury to the extensor mechanism at the level of the DIP joint.

○ **What condition is associated with osteochondritis of the upper femoral epiphysis?**

Legg-Calvé-Perthes disease.

○ **Injury to which nerve will result in a Trendelenberg limp?**

The superior gluteal nerve.

○ **What is the common name for a metacarpal fracture?**

A boxer's fracture.

○ **What is the treatment of choice for a unicameral bone cyst?**

Curettage and bone grafting.

○ *Which carpal bone is most frequently fractured?*

The scaphoid bone.

❍   **What are the typical characteristics of causalgia?**

Severe burning pain, hyperesthesia and vasomotor instability.

❍   **What is the recommended treatment for late stage torticollis?**

Operative division of the fibrotic musculofascial structures.

❍   **What is the increase in energy expenditure required to walk with an above-knee amputation prosthesis?**

100%

❍   **What are the histological characteristics of aneurysmal bone cysts?**

Cavernous spaces within fibrous tissue that lack an endothelial lining.

❍   **What is the treatment of DeQuervain's stenosing tenosynovitis after failed medical management?**

Surgical release of the first extensor compartment.

❍   **What is the appropriate management of Osgood-Schlatter disease?**

Symptomatic and conservative. Symptoms usually disappear after fusion of the tibial tubercle apophysis.

❍   **What complication is unique to fractures through the growth plate of bone?**

A bone bridge across the physis with eventual asymmetry or cessation of growth from the physis.

❍   **What benign tumor arises from chondroblasts?**

Chondromas.

❍   **What is the etiology of pseudoarthrosis?**

Continued movement at the fracture site that stimulates formation of a false joint.

❍   **What is the standard treatment for elderly patients with Garden III and IV femoral neck fractures?**

Femoral hemiarthroplasty.

❍   *What complications are associated with displaced fractures of the scaphoid?*

Avascular necrosis and nonunion.

❍   *What is the most sensitive clinical finding of compartment syndrome in an alert patient?*

Pain with passive stretch.

❍   **What is the composition of woven bone?**

Disorganized yet highly mineralized tissue.

❍   *How much blood can be stored in the thigh after a closed femur fracture?*

2 to 3 units.

○   **What is the etiology of isolated anterior cruciate ligament tears?**

Hyperextension of the knee or forceful internal rotation of the tibia on the femur.

○   **What joints are most commonly affected by osteoarthritis?**

The large weight-bearing joints (e.g., hips, knees).

○   **What are the hip-stabilizing muscles?**

The piriformis, obturator internus, gemelli and gluteus medius.

○   **What is the major cause of failure of total joint arthroplasty?**

Aseptic mechanical loosening at the interface between the bone, cement and the implant.

○   **What is the average life expectancy of prostheses used for hip and knee replacements?**

15 years.

○   **What is the proper way to transport an amputated body part to optimize its chance for replantation?**

It should be cleaned of debris, wrapped in a sterile towel moistened with sterile saline, placed in a sterile plastic bag and transported in an insulated cooler with ice water.

○   **What is the typical presentation of osteoarthritis?**

Joint pain brought on by motion and weight bearing that is relieved with rest.

BREAST PEARLS

Nothing in life is to be feared; it is only to be understood.
Marie Curie

O **What is the embryologic etiology of amastia?**

Arrest of mammary ridge development in the sixth week of fetal development.

O **What are the clinical manifestations of Poland's syndrome?**

Absence of the pectoralis major and minor muscles, malformation of the ipsilateral upper limb, unilateral amastia, hypoplasia of the ipsilateral costal cartilages, ribs and subcutaneous tissues of the chest wall and brachysyndactyly.

O **T/F: Accessory breast tissue is usually bilateral.**

True.

O **What type of nerve cell ending provides sensation to the nipple?**

Meissner's corpuscle.

O **T/F: Batson's plexus is a route of metastasis for breast cancer.**

True, vertebral veins without valves allow for metastatic "reflux" to the brain

O **T/F: Premenopausal women with node-positive breast cancer have improved survival rate with the use of adjuvant chemotherapy.**

True.

O **What is the initial treatment of tender, firm, cord mass on lateral aspect of breast?**

Mondor's disease is thrombophlebitis of superficial vein on the breast. Tx: Nsaid.

O *DCIS is found in breast mass. What is the definitive treatment?*

Lumpectomy+ RT. Radiation has been shown to dramatically reduce recurrence.
No axillary lymph node dissection.
Mastectomy may be required with combination of poor margins, high grade, and large segment of DCIS.

O **What is the sensory innervation of the breast?**

The lateral and anterior cutaneous branches of the second through sixth intercostal nerves.

O **Where are Rotter's nodes located?**

In the interpectoral region.

O **What are Level II lymph nodes?**

Those located behind the pectoralis minor muscle.

O   **Positive supraclavicular lymph nodes in breast cancer confer what stage?**

Stage IV.

O   **What is the initiating factor for ductal development?**

Estrogen.

O   **T/F: Adolescent males often experience bilateral gynecomastia.**

False; it is usually unilateral.

O   **How much radiation is delivered per mammogram?**

0.1 rads.

O   **What mammographic findings are suggestive of cancer?**

Fine, stippled calcium in an occult or suspicious lesion, architectural distortion, duct dilatation, asymmetry and fibronodular densities.

O   **What is the true-positive rate of mammography when conducted in an optimal environment?**

Greater than 90%.

O   **What percentage of patients with clinically detected breast cancer have positive axillary nodes at diagnosis?**

Greater than 50%.

O   **What percentage of patients with mammographically detected breast cancer have positive axillary nodes at diagnosis?**

Less than 20%.

O   **What is the role of MRI in detection of breast cancer?**

Its role in screening is unclear. However, it is valuable in detecting metastasis to the vertebral bodies and musculoskeletal system.

O   **What is the primary indication for ductography?**

Evaluation of bloody nipple discharge.

O   *What is the appropriate initial diagnostic procedure for identification of a palpable breast mass?*

Fine needle aspiration (FNA).

O   **What is the state-of-the-art for localizing nonpalpable breast masses?**

Mammographic needle localization.

O   **What organisms are most frequently recovered from the nipple discharge of a patient with an infected breast?**

Staphylococcus aureus and streptococci.

○ **What fungal infections most frequently affect the breast?**

Blastomycosis and sporotrichosis.

○ **What is the most common cause of fungal infections of the breast?**

Infant suckling.

○ **What are the boarders of a formal axillary dissection ?**

Latissimus Dorsi, Chest Wall, Axillary Vein; Thoracodorsal Nerve.

○ **Which nerve innervates the muscle responsible for arm adduction?**

The Thoracodorsal, which innervates the Latissimus dorsi.

○ **Which nerve is responsible for sensation to the medial aspect of arm?**

Intercostobrachial.

○ **Poland syndrome consists of what congential abnormalities?**

Hypoplastic Shoulder.
Amastia.
Absence of pectoralis muscles.

○ *What is the appropriate management of patients with Mondor's disease?*

Salicylates, warm compresses, restriction of range of motion and shoulder and brassiere support.

○ **T/F: The prognosis for breast cancer is the same for pregnant and nonpregnant women.**

True.

○ *When is fribrocystic disorder associated with an increased risk of breast cancer?*

When there is an associated dysplasia.

○ **What is the next step in management following drainage of a large, clear, fluid-filled breast cyst?**

Reassurance.

○ T/F: Male breast cancer, stage for stage, has a worse prognosis than adenocarcinoma of the breast in a female.

False, male breast cancer tends to present at a later stage, but the stage specific survival is similar to that of women.

○ *What is the appropriate treatment following drainage of a cyst that contained bloody fluid?*

Cyst excision.

○ **What is the etiology of skin dimpling in women with breast cancer?**

Glandular fibrosis and shortening of Cooper's ligaments.

○   **What is the effect of adjuvant radiotherapy following mastectomy for breast cancer?**

It decreases the local recurrence rate but does not increase survival.

○   *T/F: Atypical hyperplasia is associated with a 10-fold increased risk of breast cancer.*

False, it is approximately 4x greater though, the only finding in fibrocytic disease associated with increased CA rate.

○   **What are the characteristics of sclerosing adenosis?**

Lobulocentric changes causing distortion and enlargement of lobular units, an increased numbers of acinar structures and fibrous changes.

○   **What is the current recommended therapy for patients with Stage I and II breast cancer?**

Modified radical mastectomy (MRM) or wide local excision with axillary dissection/sentinel node biopsy and radiation therapy.

○   **What is the typical clinical presentation of ductal ectasia?**

A perimenopausal women with palpable lumpiness beneath the areola and nipple discharge.

○   **What is comedo mastitis?**

The presence of grumous, pultaceous material within dilated ducts that mimics comedo carcinoma and is caused by ductal ectasia.

○   **T/F: Gynecomasia in a male is associated with an increased rate of future breast cancer.**

False.

○   *What is the characteristic gross appearance of a fibroadenoma?*

Sharp circumscription with smooth boundaries and a glistening, white cut surface.

○   **T/F: Fibroadenomas are invariably related to estrogen sensitivity.**

True.

○   **What is the most frequently employed hormonal manipulation in patients with breast cancer?**

Estrogen withdrawal (tamoxifen).

○   **What is the most common initial site of metastases in breast cancer?**

The bone.

○   **How much toes tamoxifen therapy reduce the incidence of recurrent breast cancer when used for 5 years?**

50%.

○   **Do premenopausal women, with node positive breast cancer benefit from radiation therapy after receiving wide excision with negative margins, axillary dissection, and chemotherapy?**

Yes, local recurrence rate in this patient subgroup is reduced from 30% to 15%

○ *What is the most common cause of bloody nipple discharge?*

Intraductal papilloma.

○ **What percentage of cancer-related deaths in women are related to breast cancer?**
20%.

○ **What type of breast cancer most frequently presents with a palpable mass?**

Infiltrating ductal carcinoma.

○ **What primary ductal carcinoma presents with a chronic, erythematous, oozing and eczematoid rash involving the nipple and areola?**

Paget's disease of the breast.

○ **T/F: Use of combined oral contraceptives increases the risk of breast cancer.**

False.

○ *What is the initial treatment for inflammatory breast cancer?*

Chemotherapy, followed by surgical excision and XRT.

○ **Inflammatory breast carcinoma is a variant of which type of breast cancer?**

Infiltrating ductal carcinoma.

○ **What is the most common primary sarcoma of the breast?**

Cystosarcoma (phylloides tumor).

○ **What percentage of cystosarcomas are malignant?**

10%.

○ **Does Tamoxifen have a role in DCIS?**

Yes, it reduces recurrence of DCIS.

○ **T/F: Women with a history of ovarian cancer are at increased risk of breast cancer.**

True.

○ **What is the average 5-year survival for Stage IV breast cancer?**

Less than 20%.

○ **What is the recurrence rate of breast cancer in women with recurrent lymph node involvement?**

50 to 75%.

○ *What is the appropriate treatment for a patient with a small, localized phyllodes tumor?*

Local excision without lymp node biopsy.

○ **What is the median survival for women with untreated breast cancer?**

35 months from the onset of symptoms.

○ **What percentage of breast carcinomas occur in men?**

1%.

○ **What is the most common cause of death in women with breast cancer following mastectomy?**

Metastatic disease.

○ **What is the most important prognostic indicator for recurrent breast cancer and metastatic disease in women with breast cancer?**

Nodal status at the time of initial diagnosis.

○ **What is the average age at diagnosis of invasive breast cancer?**

60 years.

○ **What percentage of invasive lobular carcinomas are estrogen sensitive?**

90%.

○ **What is the distinguishing feature of LCIS?**

Cytoplasmic mucoid globules.

○ *What is the medical treatment of radiation mastitis?*

Trenal (pentoxifylline).

PLASTIC AND RECONSTRUCTIVE SURGERY PEARLS

Do not resist growing old —— many are denied the privilege.
Anonymous

○ **What are the disadvantages of meshed skin grafts?**

They contract more than sheet grafts and have an inferior aesthetic result.

○ **What type of incision(s) should be used on skin overlying joints?**

Oblique or transverse incisions.

○ **What are the complications of excessive tension across a wound?**

Delayed wound healing and a wide scar.

○ **What is the second phase of skin graft contraction?**

Contraction of the recipient bed.

○ **How might spinal or epidural anesthesia be a disadvantage in patients undergoing lipectomy or liposuction?**

The anticipated volume of aspirate may exceed 1 liter and estimation of the patient's volume status may be complicated by the sympathetic blockade.

○ *What suture material loses its strength within 7 days?*

Plain gut.

○ **The bipedicle mucoperiosteal flap is based upon what vessels?**

The greater palatine vessels.

○ **What is the difference between primary and secondary skin graft contraction?**

Primary contraction refers to the immediate shrinkage that occurs after removal from the donor site. Secondary contraction is the phenomenon that occurs as the graft heals.

○ **What is the most important factor in minimizing hyperpigmentation of skin grafts?**

Protection from UV light for a full year postoperatively.

○ **What are the indications for dermal overgrafting?**

Unstable, depressed or hypertrophied scars, unstable or hyperpigmented skin grafts, large pigmented nevi, radiation damage and tattoos.

○   **What is the appropriate ratio of the long and short axes for elliptical incisions?**

4:1.

○   **What complication will occur if the above ratio is not met?**

A dog-ear deformity.

○   **What is the single most reliable test of graft viability?**

Examination by an experienced physician.

○   **What is the chance of producing a cleft-lipped child when one parent is affected?**

4%.

○   **When does irreversible ischemia of peripheral nerves occur?**

Within 8 hours of warm ischemia.

○   **When is return of sensation after skin grafting considered maximal?**

After 2 years.

○   **How long can skin grafts be stored when banked in saline-soaked gauze sponges at 4° Celsius?**

Up to 21 days.

○   **What is the single most important factor in the management of contaminated wounds?**

Debridement of devitalized tissue.

○   **What is the most important factor in the aesthetic outcome of lip reconstruction?**

Alignment of the vermillion border.

○   **What are the boundaries of a unilateral cleft of the primary palate?**

From the incisor foramen anteriorly, between the canine and adjacent incisor to the lip.

○   **What is a V-Y advancement?**

Closure of a rectangular defect by incising an adjacent triangle of tissue and advancing it into the defect.

○   **What is the appropriate treatment for a patient with a Stage III decubitus ulcer?**

Sharp debridement of devitalized and infected tissue and conservative management.

○   **What tissue is most sensitive to hypoxia?**

The vascular endothelium.

❍ **What is the most appropriate type of microvascular anastamosis if there is a discrepancy of lumen size greater than 2:1?**

An end-to-end anastamosis.

❍ **What is the success rate for free-tissue transfers?**

Greater than 90%.

❍ **The midline forehead flap is based on what vessels?**

The supratrochlear vessels.

❍ *T/F: Split-thickness skin grafts (STSG) contract more than full-thickness skin grafts (FTSG).*

True.

❍ **What are the recommended margins for excision of basal cell skin cancers?**

5 mm.

❍ **What is the characteristic nasal deformity in a child with a unilateral cleft lip?**

Inferior and posterior displacement of the alar cartilage on the cleft side.

❍ **What percentage of incompletely excised basal cell cancers will recur?**

One-third.

❍ **T/F: Tissue expanders increase the vascularity of skin.**

True.

❍ **What is the rule of 10's for guiding the timing of definitive cleft lip repair?**

Lip repair is performed when the child has reached a weight of 10 pounds, is 10 weeks old and has a hematocrit greater than 10 mg/dl.

❍ **What is the appropriate ratio of crystalloid infusion to fat removal in suction lipectomy?**

3:1.

❍ **What is the embryologic etiology of cleft lip?**

Failure of the nasolabial and nasolateral processes to fuse and/or failure of mesodermal migration.

❍ **What is the primary palate?**

The lip, alveolus and the hard palate to the incisor foramen.

❍ **What type of skin graft is most appropriate for resurfacing the upper eyelid?**

FTSG.

❍ **What type of flap is most appropriate in the treatment of osteomyelitis?**

A muscle flap.

❍   **What is the blood supply of a random flap?**

The dermal and subdermal plexuses.

❍   **Where are basal cell cancers most likely to recur after adequate treatment?**

Around the orbits, nose and ears.

❍   **What histologic characteristic of recurrent basal cell cancers has prognostic significance?**

Irregularity in the peripheral palisade.

❍   **What is the most frequently utilized flap for head and neck reconstruction?**

The deltopectorial flap.

❍   **What is the estimated risk for developing a new basal or squamous cell cancer at 3 and 5 years?**

35% and 50%, respectively.

❍   **The dermis primarily contains what type(s) of collagen?**

Type I (80%) and Type III (15%).

❍   **What is the reported ratio of basal cell to squamous cell cancer in the United States?**

4:1.

❍   **What are the predictors of tumor recurrence in squamous cell cancer of the skin?**

Degree of cellular differentiation, depth of tumor invasion and perineural invasion.

❍   **The greater omentum axial flap is based on what vessels?**

Either the right or the left gastroepiploic artery.

❍   **Squamous cell cancers in which areas of the body are prone to metastasis?**

Scalp, ears, nostrils and extremities.

❍   **What type of flap rotates about its axis to fill an adjacent defect?**

A transposition flap.

❍   **What is the most appropriate donor site for grafting the skin of the face?**

Postauricular.

❍   *What are the risk factors for melanoma?*

Fair complexion, red hair, greater than 20 nevi on the body, previous diagnosis of melanoma in the individual or first degree relative and immunodeficiency.

❍   **What tissues are included in the posterior thigh fasciocutaneous flap?**

The fascia lata, subcutaneous skin and tissue and the descending branch of the inferior gluteal artery.

❍   *What is the recommended excisional margin for a 3 cm melanoma?*

2 cm.

❍   **What is the treatment of choice for a subungal melanoma?**

Amputation at the interphalangeal joint of the thumb and the distal interphalangeal joint of the finger or at the metatarsal-phalangeal joint of the toe.

❍   **What is the most appropriate donor site for grafting the skin of the hand?**

The anticubital crease or the inner aspect of the arm.

❍   **What finding on inspection of a flap indicates venous thrombosis?**

Development of a sharp line of color demarcation.

❍   **What is the clinical definition of ptosis of the breast?**

When the nipple is below the level of the inframammary crease.

❍   **What is the incidence of skip metastasis in melanoma?**

2%.

❍   *What factor, other than tumor thickness, predictss regional metastasis in melanoma?*

Ulceration.

❍   **What are the limiting factors in the use of muscle flaps?**

The size of the muscle and the length of its vascular pedicle.

❍   **What is the risk of melanomatous transformation of giant congenital nevi?**

14%.

❍   **What process allows survival of skin grafts in the first 48 hours?**

Plasmatic imbibition.

❍   **What are the indications for therapeutic intervention in a patient with a hemangioma?**

Obstruction of the eye, airway, oropharynx or auditory canal, large ulcerated lesions with secondary hemorrhage or infection, Kasabach-Merritt syndrome and hemangiomas of the head and neck that are sources of psychosocial trauma.

❍   **What is meant by inoscultation with regard to skin grafts?**

The process by which vascular buds from the recipient bed make contact with capillaries within the graft.

❍   **What are the components of Sturge-Weber syndrome?**

A facial port-wine stain over at least the first and second divisions of the trigeminal nerve, leptomeningeal venous malformations and mental retardation.

❍   **What osteotomies are made in a LeFort III facial advancement?**

Osteotomies of the nasofrontal junction, floor of the orbit, lateral maxilla and pterygomaxillary fissure for anterior advancement of the midface.

○   **What is the most common cause of acquired maxillomandibular disproportion?**

Trauma.

○   **What is the diagnostic test of choice for orbital fractures?**

CT scan with axial and coronal views.

○   *What type of cancer is red or purple cutaneous nodule, and neuroendocrine tumor staining for enolase and nuerofilament?*

Merkel cell carcinoma.

○   **Hidadrenitis involves what type of glands?**

Apocrine glands.

○   **What is the most common skin cancer?**

Basal cell Ca.

○   **What is the difference between Keloid and Hypertrophic scar?**

Keloid extends beyond wound margins and is associated with failure of collagen breakdown and increased collagen production. Hypertrophic scar does not extend beyond the margins.

○   **What is the treatment of choice for patients with unstable mandibular fractures?**

Open reduction and internal fixation (ORIF).

○   **T/F: A fracture through the body of the mandible that courses obliquely and anteriorly from anterior to posterior is classified as unfavorable.**

True.

○   **What is the best approach for repair of naso-orbital-ethmoid (NOE) fractures?**

A bicoronal incision.

○   **What is the typical presentation of a patient with a fracture of the zygomaticomaxillary complex?**

Enophthalmus, diplopia (particularly on upward gaze) and opacification of the maxillary sinus.

○   **What patients require a forced duction test?**

Those with orbital floor fractures.

○   **What is a LeFort I maxillary fracture?**

A maxillary fracture that extends from the piriform aperture laterally to the pterygomaxillary fissure.

○   **T/F: Hearing is usually impaired in patients with microtia.**

True.

○ **What lip defects may be closed primarily?**

Defects of up to one-third of the lower lip and one-fourth of the upper lip.

○ **What layers of the eyelid require re-approximation in through-and-through lacerations?**

The conjunctiva and tarsal plate, the orbiculeris oculi muscle and the skin.

○ **What is the most common cause of acquired ptosis?**

Dysfunction of the oculomotor nerve or sympathetic chain, usually due to trauma.

○ **What are the characteristics of an immature hemangioma?**

They have a raised bright red color, may not be present at birth, become evident in the neonatal period, grow rapidly and usually involute spontaneously by 7 years of age.

○ **What functional problems result from facial nerve paralysis?**

Exposure keratitis, oral incompetence, abnormal speech, facial asymmetry and profound diminution of facial expression.

○ **What is the most common lymphatic malformation found in the head and neck?**

A cystic hygroma.

○ **What are the possible benefits of breast reconstruction?**

1. Improved body image.
2. Preservation of feminine identity.
3. Elimination of external prostheses.
4. Lessened psychosocial impact of mastectomy.

○ **What complications are associated with breast reconstruction with a tissue expander or implant?**

Hematoma, infection, exposure of the implant and capsular contraction.

○ **What is the primary blood supply for a transverse rectus abdominus musculocutaenous (TRAM) flap?**

The superior epigastric vessels.

○ **What are the complications of macromastia?**

Back pain, brassiere strap furrowing, skin irritation in the inframammary fold and breast pain.

○ **What are the possible complications of breast reduction procedures?**

A long scar that is difficult to hide, hematoma, fat necrosis, nipple necrosis and hypertrophic scar formation.

○ **What is the most common complication of breast augmentation?**

Capsular contraction.

○ **T/F: Women with silicone breast implants have an increased incidence of collagen vascular disease.**

False.

○   **What is the most common flap for a greater trochanter pressure sore?**

The tensor fascia lata myocutaneous flap.

○   **What are the preferred flaps for proximal one-third tibial wounds?**

Gastrocnemius and soleus flaps.

○   **What are the most important factors in choosing immediate versus delayed breast reconstruction?**

The vascular supply and degree of tension of the skin flap.

○   **What is the most appropriate treatment for distal one-third tibial wounds?**

Free-tissue transfer.

○   **What is lymphedema tardum?**

Congenital lymphedema that presents after the age of 35 years.

NEUROSURGERY PEARLS

We know the human brain is a device to keep the ears from grating on one another.

Peter De Vries

○ *What are the scoring criteria for the glascow-coma score?*

Motor *6-follows commands; 5 withdraws from painful stimuli; 4 localizes pain; 3 flexion posturing; 2 extension posturing; 1-flaccid.*

Verbal *5-appropriate; 4 Confused; 3 Inappropriate; 2 Incomprehensible sounds; 1 No vocalizing.*

Eyes *4 spontaneous; 3 open to voice; 2 open to painful stimuli; 1 do not open.*

Total score 10 or less - intubation.
Total score 8 or less with head trauma - ICP monitor.

○ **What is the most common cause of cerebrospinal fluid (CSF) leaks?**

Basilar skull fractures.

○ **What therapy should be used for a patient with hemophilia A who has suffered a traumatic brain injury?**

Cryoprecipitate.

○ **What is the diagnostic yield of lumbar punctures for organisms causing brain abscess?**

20%.

○ **What is considered a safe time interval for acutely re-opening an internal carotid artery occlusion?**

6 hours.

○ **How long should seizure prophylaxis be administered after severe traumatic brain injury?**

7 days.

○ **What is the minimum systemic arterial pressure required to maintain cerebral perfusion?**

At least 50 mm Hg.

○ **What measures assist in decreasing intracranial pressure (ICP) and increasing systemic arterial pressure?**

Elevation of the head of the bed to 30°, intermittent drainage of CSF, hyperventilation and fluid restriction.

○ **What is the incidence of postoperative meningitis after craniotomy?**

0.3 to 0.5%.

O   **What are the neurological signs of cerebellar abscesses?**

Ipsilateral horizontal nystagmus, ipsilateral dysmetria and ataxia.

O   **T/F: The presence of low signal intensity in the center of an enhancing lesion differentiates tumors from abscesses.**

False.

O   **What is the appropriate empiric antibiotic therapy for a spinal epidural abscess?**

A penicillinase-resistant penicillin (e.g., nafcillin and oxacillin).

O   **What radiographic feature of the vertebral body endplates is useful in differentiating metastatic lesions from infectious osteomyelitis?**

Tumors tend to respect the endplates, whereas infections often destroy the endplate and involve the disc space.

O   **What ECG changes are associated with brain injuries?**

Sinus tachycardia, QT-interval prolongation, pan-precordial T-wave inversion, QRS-widening and ventricular tachycardia.

O   **What are the clinical characteristics of DIC associated with severe brain injury?**

Prolongation of the prothrombin time (PT), decreased fibrinogen level and elevation of fibrin split products.

O   *Head injury can produce both Diabetes Insipidus and Syndrome of Inappropriate Diurectic Hormone. Compare and contrast the two.*

DI=High Na, high serum osm, high urine output, low urine specific gravity.
SIADH=Low Na, low serum osm, low urine out put , high urine specific gravity.

O   *What is more deadly a epidural or subdural hematoma?*

Subdural has 50% mortality.

O   **Which cerebral artery is commonly injured in the setting of lateral transtentorial herniation?**

The calcarine branch of the posterior cerebral artery.

O   **What are the clinical features of injury of Kernohan's notch?**

Uncal herniation causing ipsilateral pupil dilation and ipsilateral hemiparesis from contralateral compression of the cerebral peduncle against the contralateral tentorium.

O   **What are pontine pupils?**

Pinpoint but reactive pupils secondary to injury of the sympathetic fibers descending through the tegmentum.

O   **What are the most common causes of persistent sequelae after minor head trauma?**

Residua of organic brain damage, quest for secondary gain and psychological reaction to the injury.

O   **What are the clinical features of traumatic CSF rhinorrhea?**

Anosmia or meningitis.

○ **What is the incidence of epilepsy in patients with traumatic intracranial hematomas?**

As high as 30 to 36%.

○ **What are the most common causes of delayed increase in neurological deficit after traumatic spinal cord injury?**

Post-traumatic syrinx formation or enlargement and persistent spinal cord compression.

○ **What percentage of patients with anterior cord syndromes regain the ability to walk without assistance?**

Less than 50%.

○ *What diagnosis must be investigated in a patient presenting with pulsating exophthalmos?*

Carotid-cavernous fistula.

○ **What artery may be injured during repair of a posterior communicating artery aneurysm?**

The anterior choroidal artery.

○ **Ossification of the posterior longitudinal ligament is most common in what ethnic group?**

East Asians.

○ **T/F: Patients with severe traumatic brain injury should be routinely hyperventilated.**

False.

○ **What is the most common primary malignant brain tumor?**

Glioblastoma multiforme (GBM).

○ **What clinical features are strongly associated with increased survival after spinal cord compression by tumor?**

The ability to walk and urinary continence.

○ **What surgical procedure for trigeminal neuralgia has the lowest incidence of facial anesthesia?**

Microvascular decompression.

○ **What is the median postoperative survival for patients with GBM who do not receive radiation therapy following surgery?**

4 months.

○ **What are the most frequent sites of hemorrhage from carotid bifurcation aneurysms?**

The frontal lobe, temporal lobe and basal ganglia.

○ **What is the risk of cerebral infarction in the first 5 years following posterior circulation transient ischemic attacks (TIAs)?**

35%.

○ **What segment of the vertebral artery is most often injured in a dissection?**

The segment between the second cervical vertebra and the occiput.

❍   **What segment of the superior sagittal sinus may be occluded without clinical findings?**

The anterior one-third.

❍   **What are the most common presenting symptoms of a glomus jugulare tumor?**

Hearing loss and pulsatile tinnitus.

❍   **How long after spinal radiation can transverse myelitis persist?**

6 months to 5 years.

❍   **What dose of radiation is used in interstitial brachytherapy?**

1 to 2 rad/minute.

❍   *What surgical procedure may produce Nelson's syndrome?*

Adrenalectomy.

❍   *What is the implication of decerbrate posturing?*

Brain stem compression or injury.

❍   **What is the most common tumor of the primary posterior fossa in adults?**

Hemangioblastoma.

❍   **What is the peak incidence of cerebellar astrocytomas?**

In the middle of the first decade.

❍   **What is the most common presenting symptom in a child with a brainstem glioma?**

Gait disturbance.

❍   **What is the most appropriate treatment for a patient with a choroid plexus papilloma?**

Total surgical excision.

❍   *What are the most common initial symptoms in patients with acoustic neuromas?*

Tinnitus, hearing loss and unsteadiness.

❍   **What is the average 5-year survival for patients with infratentorial, intracranial ependymomas who undergo surgery and radiation therapy?**

90%.

❍   *What symptoms, related to lumbar disc herniation, are indications for emergency surgery?*

Urinary retention, perineal numbness and motor weakness of more than a single nerve root.

❍   **What are the potential causes of delayed neurological deterioration in patients with intracranial aneurysm rupture?**

Bleeding, vasospasm, hydrocephalus and seizures.

❍   **What is the most common location for a posterior fossa aneurysm?**

At the basilar bifurcation.

❍   **What bacteria is most commonly associated with mycotic aneurysms?**

Streptococcus.

❍   **What are the most common clinical problems seen at the initial presentation of a patient with an intracranial arteriovenous malformation?**

Seizures and hemorrhage.

❍   **Which type of craniosynostosis is the most common?**

Scaphocephaly.

❍   **What syndromes can be seen on presentation in a patient with a Type 1 Chiari malformation?**

Foramen magnum compression, central cord syndrome and cerebellar syndrome.

❍   **What is a clay shoveler's fracture?**

Avulsion of a spinous process (usually C7).

❍   **What is the most common type of odontoid fracture?**

Type II (fracture through the base of the dens).

❍   **What is the most likely diagnosis in a patient presenting with symptoms of neurogenic claudication?**

Lumbar spinal stenosis.

❍   **What spinal abnormality is commonly seen in patients with rheumatoid arthritis?**

Atlanto-axial subluxation.

❍   **What signs and symptoms characterize benign intracranial hypertension?**

Pseudotumor cerebri, headache, blurred vision, pulsatile tinnitus, vertigo, hearing loss and papilledema.

❍   **What are the disadvantages of using technetium scans to monitor therapy for narcotizing otitis externa?**

It reflects osteoblastic activity and bone remodeling but is not specific for osteomyelitis. It also has poor spatial resolution and may remain positive long after clinical resolution.

❍   **What blood vessel is frequently found at the internal auditory meatus?**

A loop of the anterior internal carotid artery.

❍   **Why is facial electroneurography (ENG) an unreliable prognostic indicator more than 3 weeks after the onset of facial paralysis?**

Asynchronous discharge from regenerating nerve fibers produces a diminished response.

○   *What are the symptomes of anterior spinal artery syndrome?*

Loss of bilateral motor, pain and temperature loss.
Position and light touch intac.

○   *What is Brown Sequard syndrome?*

Penetrating trauma with 1/2 cord transaction.
Loss of ipsilateral motor and contralateral pain and temp

○   *What is Central Cord syndrome?*

Usually a MVA of elderly pts with hyperextension injury.
Bilateral loss of upper extremity motor pain and temp. The legs retain function.

○   *When is surgery required for skull fx?*

Open or depressed skull fracture.

○   **What are the major sources of brain abscesses?**

Direct extension from middle ear, mastoid and sinus infections, hematogenous spread and trauma.

○   *Bilateral facial paralysis associated with progressive ascending motor neuropathy of the lower extremities and elevated CSF protein is characteristic of what clinical entity?*

Guillian-Barré syndrome.

○   **How would you grade facial nerve function in a patient with facial asymmetry at rest, incomplete eye closure and minimal motion of the mouth with maximal effort?**

House Grade V.

○   **In the tonotopic organization of the cochlea, where are the low frequencies located?**

At the cochlear apex.

○   **Following incus erosion, ossicular reconstruction using the intact and mobile stapes can be performed with what prostheses?**

Partial ossicular reconstruction prosthesis (POP or PORP), incus prosthesis (e.g., Wehrs) or autografts carved from residual incus.

○   **T/F: ENG detection of horizontal nystagmus that spontaneously changes direction while the patient lies in the left lateral position is most consistent with labyrinthitis.**

False.

○   **T/F: Early detection of labyrinthitis ossificans is a contraindication to cochlear implantation.**

False.

○   **What ENG criterion is used to recommend surgical decompression of the facial nerve after blunt temporal bone trauma?**

Greater than 90% degeneration within 2 weeks.

○ **Recurrent facial paralysis, facial edema, furrowed tongue and cheilitis are consistent with what diagnosis?**

Melkersson-Rosenthal syndrome.

○ **What are the characteristics of Gradenigo's syndrome?**

Petrous apicitis, diplopia, otorrhea and retro-orbital pain.

○ **What are the imaging characteristics of a cholesterol granuloma of the petrous apex on MRI?**

Hyperintense on T1- and T2- weighted images.

○ **What are the embryologic origins of the stapes?**

The superstructure is derived from the second branchial arch and the footplate originates from the otic mesenchyme.

○ **Bill's bar separates what anatomic structures?**

The facial nerve from the superior vestibular nerve.

○ *What organism is associated with necrotizing otitis externa?*

Pseudomonas aeruginosa.

○ **What is the function of the spiral ganglion cells in the cochlea?**

They are the bipolar first-order neurons that contact the hair cells and form the cochlear nerve.

○ **T/F: Barbiturates minimize intracellular edema.**

True.

○ **What is the mechanism of action of the otolithic organs?**

The saccule and utricle are stimulated by linear acceleration in 3 planes and by static tilt (gravitational acceleration).

○ **T/F: A narrow internal auditory canal is a contraindication for cochlear implantation.**

True.

○ *Bilateral acoustic neuromas are found in what clinical entity?*

Neurofibromatosis II.

○ **What surgical approaches to acoustic neuroma resection can spare hearing?**

The middle fossa and retrosigmoid/suboccipital approach.

○ **What nonglial neoplasm arises from the meningothelial cells of the arachnoid villi?**

Meningiomas.

❍   **T/F: Electrocochleography is the study of choice for patients with episodic vertigo and congenital deafness.**

False.

❍   **In a child with bilateral congenital aural atresia, how is normal sensorineural hearing confirmed in the ear to be operated on first?**

Detection of an ipsilateral wave I on bone conduction ABR.

❍   **What is the typical physical finding in patients with a congenital cholesteatoma?**

A white middle ear mass beneath an intact tympanic membrane.

❍   **T/F: Most acoustic neuromas are inherited on chromosome 22.**

False.

❍   **What radiologic findings are characteristic of Histiocytosis X?**

Single or multiple sharply circumscribed osteolytic lesions, most frequently found on the skull.

❍   **What is the most common tumor of the middle ear?**

A glomus tumor.

❍   **What is the most common site of origin of glomus tympanicum tumors?**

Jacobson's nerve.

❍   **Which intracranial tumors are radiosensitive?**

Pituitary adenomas, craniopharyngiomas and certain tumors of the pineal region.

❍   **What are the histologic features of acoustic neuroma?**

Spindle cells in short interlacing fascicles with whole, ring or palisading nuclei. Alternating regions of Antoni A (compact spindle cells) and Antoni B (hypocellular areas) is found. The tumor is S-100 positive.

❍   **What are the histologic features of glomus tumors?**

Nests of chief cells with surrounding fibrovascular stroma, sustentacular cells at the periphery of the cell nests that are S-100 positive and neurosecretory granules in the chief cells. In addition, the chief cells are positive on immunohistochemistry for chromogranin, synaptophysin and neuron-specific enolase neurofilaments.

❍   *How long can a CSF leak, without signs of infection, be observed?*

Up to 14 days.

❍   **What is the primary treatment for erysipelas involving the ear?**

Oral or intravenous antistreptococcal antibiotics.

❍   **What is the speech reception threshold?**

The lowest intensity level at which a person can correctly identify 50% of spoken words.

O   **What type of tympanogram is associated with ossicular discontinuity?**

Type AD.

O   **T/F: The afferent fibers of the auditory nerve innervate the inner hair cells.**

True.

O   **What are the intraoperative options for a mobilized stapedial footplate during attempted stapedectomy?**

Place an osteotomy in the promontory edge of the oval window and pass a small hook to remove the footplate, laser stapedotomy or allow the footplate to correct itself and attempt stapedectomy at a later date.

O   **What is the appropriate treatment for vasospasm in patients with a subarachnoid hemorrhage?**

Relative hypertension, relative hypovolemia and calcium channel blockers.

O   **When does denervation atrophy of muscles become irreversible?**

After 12 to 15 months.

O   **What radiographic findings are associated with Type I Arnold-Chiari malformation?**

Downward herniation of the cerebellar tonsils through the foramen magnum.

O   **A patient with known HIV infection presents with seizures and 2 ring-enhancing brain lesions. What is the most likely diagnosis?**

Toxoplasmosis or a CNS lymphoma.

O   **A transplant recipient presents with a ring-enhancing lesion and seizures. What is the most likely diagnosis?**

An infectious abscess.

O   **A patient with a history of lung cancer presents with a seizure and a ring-enhancing lesion on CT of the brain. Examination reveals a new heart murmur in an otherwise normal patient with normal vital signs and no history of fever. What is the most likely diagnosis?**

Bacterial endocarditis.

O   **A child presents with headache, lethargy, erythema and forehead tenderness. After a CT of the brain, what treatment should be undertaken?**

Drainage of the infected paranasal sinuses.

O   **A 22 year old female presents 2 weeks postpartum with a severe headache and lethargy. CT scan shows the empty delta sign with some enhancement of the tentorium and cortical surface. What is the most likely diagnosis?**

Sagittal sinus thrombosis.

O   *What criteria must be met to establish the diagnosis of the Syndrome of Inappropriate Anti-Diuretic Hormone (SIADH)?*

A low serum sodium and euvolemia.

O   *What is the treatment of choice for patients with SIADH?*

DDAVP.

O   **An infant presents with a dimple over his nasion. You notice a drop of fluid in the dimple. What is the next step in the management?**

MRI and neurosurgical consult for possible exploration.

O   **What is the most common congenital vascular abnormality of the CNS?**

Intracranial aneurysms.

O   **Following correction of a ventral abdominal hernia the patient develops meralgia and paresthesia. What complication has he suffered?**

Lateral femoral cutaneous nerve impingement.

O   *What finding is present in all types of subdural hematomas?*

A decreased level of consciousness out of proportion to the observed focal neurological deficit.

O   *What are the significant differences between Lambert-Eaton (LE) syndrome and myasthenia gravis (MG)?*

LE is associated with lung carcinoma and synaptic blockade occurs at the pre-synaptic calcium channels, impeding the release of muscle acetylcholine. In addition, LE is manifested by muscle strengthening with repetition, as opposed to fatigue with repetition in MG.

O   **What are the hallmarks of Grade IV GBM?**

Necrosis, neovascular proliferation, extensive mitosis and pleomorphism.

O   **What do neurofibromatosis, tuberous sclerosis and von Hippel-Lindau disease have in common?**

These are phakomatoses, a group of hereditary syndromes with neural, ocular and cutaneous manifestations.

O   **When should a child born with an open myelomeningocele undergo repair?**

Emergently; to prevent infection and resultant meningitis.

O   **What is the goal of a myelomeningocele repair?**

To reconstitute the normal anatomic barriers and repair the dural cutaneous fistula.

O   **What is the hallmark of the Chiari II malformation?**

Herniation of the cerebellar tonsils and inferior cerebellar vermis through the foramen magnum.

O   **Evaluation of a child reveals scoliosis and a hairy dimple above the gluteal crease. With further questioning he admits to back discomfort. The mother reports that the child has a persistent history of enuresis. What is the most appropriate diagnostic test?**

MRI of the lumbosacral spine.

O   **What tumors most commonly metastasize to the spine?**

Lymphoma, breast, prostate and kidney.

○ *A patient presents with a third nerve palsy and recent episode of excruciating headache. What is the most likely diagnosis?*

Posterior communicating artery aneurysm.

○ *A 54 year old male presents with a sudden severe headache. CT scan of the brain is normal. What is the next step in management?*

Lumbar puncture.

○ **What symptoms are associated with a grade 4 subarachnoid hemorrhage?**

Stupor, hemiparesis and posturing.

○ **Your patient develops new onset headache 1 week after presenting with subarachnoid hemorrhage and having had a cerebral aneurysm clipped. You are concerned about the development of cerebral vasospasm. What is the appropriate management?**

Maintain a mean blood pressure greater than 90 mm Hg, systolic blood pressure between 150 and 200 mm Hg, CVP less than 8 mm Hg, PAWP greater than 12 mm Hg and a hematocrit of 33%.

○ *A 35 year old trauma patient presents with quadriplegia. After resuscitation and full evaluation revealing no other injuries, the systolic blood pressure falls to 80 mm Hg. What is the appropriate intervention at this time?*

IV fluid followed by pressor support and invasive monitoring of the volume status.

○ **Why is there a higher incidence of complete neurologic loss with thoracic fractures than with cervical or lumbar fractures?**

The thoracic spinal canal has the least cross-sectional area for the spinal cord, thus, allowing less room for movement of the cord. Furthermore, since the thoracic spine is so strong, a thoracic spine injury is the result of a tremendous force. In addition, the blood supply to the thoracic cord has a more of a water-shed distribution than the other regions.

○ **Why are spinal injuries of the lumbar region more likely to have neurologic recovery than injuries to other regions of the spine?**

The neurologic compromise in the lumbar region is a result of cauda equina or lumbosacral nerve root injury, not spinal cord injury.

○ *What is the physiologic difference between epidural and subdural hematomas as seen on an axial CT scan?*

Epidural hematomas are lens-shaped because spread of the hemorrhage is contained by the tight adherence of the dura to the skull, while subdural hematomas are more concave.

○ **What is the significance of a fracture through the posterior table of the frontal sinus?**

There is potential communication between a contaminated space (the sinus) and the intracranial contents that can lead to a CSF leak or meningitis. Furthermore, significant disturbance of the sinus contours with entrapment of the sinus mucosa can lead to mucoceles.

○ **A young child is brought in for follow-up after a minor, recent fall. The parents point out a large area of fluctuance under his scalp. What is the appropriate management?**

Reassurance and follow-up.

❍   **A patient presents with rhinorrhea after recent head trauma. What is the most specific test for a CSF leak?**

Beta 2-transferrin.

❍   **T/F: Excessive hyperventilation in a patient with a head injury may cause brain ischemia and edema.**

True.

❍   *What is cerebral perfusion pressure (CPP) and what does it signify?*

CPP = MAP - ICP, where MAP equals mean arterial pressure. CPP represents the pressure required to push blood from the arterial tree to the venous tree in the intracranial space. If CPP is inadequate, the brain tissue will be underperfused.

❍   *You stabilize a multiple trauma victim whose injuries include mild head injury, scalp lacerations and a femur fracture. The next morning you note a new right hemiparesis, confusion and petechiae on his chest and in his conjunctivae. His oxygen saturation has dropped to the low 90's and his urine output is declining. What is the most likely diagnosis?*

Fat embolism.

❍   *A multiple trauma patient presents with a deteriorating level of consciousness, a dilated right pupil and left hemiparesis. He is hypotensive and has a grossly positive DPL. The patient is rushed to the operating room for exploratory laparotomy. When and how should his head injury be addressed?*

A separate team should place a right temporal fossa burr hole as the laparotomy proceeds.

❍   **What is Kernohan's Notch syndrome?**

A phenomenon in the setting of uncal herniation where temporal lobe herniation displaces the brainstem against the opposite tentorial edge (Kernohan's notch) and causes symptoms of contralateral brainstem injury and ipsilateral hemiparesis.

❍   **During the evacuation of a temporal epidural hematoma you are unable to control bleeding from the middle meningeal artery. What is the appropriate next step?**

Place a sterile toothpick in the foramen spinosum (where the middle meningeal artery enters after branching from the maxillary artery of the external carotid).

❍   **The trigeminal nerve supplies innervation to what muscles?**

The muscles of mastication (temporalis, masseter and medial and lateral pterygoid muscles).

❍   *Deviation of the tongue to the side indicates injury to what nerve?*

The ipsilateral hypoglossal nerve.

❍   **Modern trauma facilities usually feature a CT scanner as an integral part of the evaluation. Barring the cost, why do these facilities not utilize MRI for such emergent use?**

MRI typically requires a longer scan time and the patient must be completely stable.

❍   **What is the mortality rate for a patient with a Glasgow Coma Scale of 5?**

Greater than 50%.

○   **What is the difference between a communicating and a non-communicating hydrocephalus?**

A communicating hydrocephalus communicates with all of the ventricles. In a non-communicating hydrocephalus, the fourth ventricle is isolated from the dilated third and lateral ventricles.

○   **What is the physiologic basis for the difference in communication versus non-communicating hydrocephalus?**

The non-communicating form causes an obstruction to CSF flow. The obstruction in the communicating hydrocephalus is in the extra-ventricular subarachnoid space.

○   **Why does an adult with acute hydrocephalus secondary to an aneurysmal subarachnoid hemorrhage or traumatic intraventricular hemorrhage deteriorate rapidly, while a newborn with hydrocephalus from intraventricular hemorrhage appears relatively stable?**

The newborn's head is an elastic container due to the unfused skull plates, while the adult's head is a rigid closed box.

○   **T/F: Most spinal cord tumors are extradural.**

True.

○   **What is the most common type of brain tumor?**

Gliomas.

○   **You are called to consult on a child in the emergency room with abdominal discomfort, a 2-day history of nausea and vomiting and a palpable abdominal mass. There is no history of fever and bowel sounds are within normal limits. The only significant history is that of a congenital hydrocephalus previously treated with placement of a ventriculo-peritoneal shunt. The patient is cooperative but uncomfortable and has no peritoneal signs. Physical exam reveals a palpable mass in the right lower quadrant. What is the most likely diagnosis?**

An intraabdominal pseudocyst associated with an indolent VP shunt infection.

○   **What is the most appropriate diagnostic test for the above patient?**

An abdominal ultrasound or CT scan of the abdomen.

○   **Your neurosurgical colleague requests your assistance with a patient with post-surgical abdominal pain and continued nausea and emesis. The patient is an obese young adult that just underwent replacement of a ventriculo-peritoneal shunt that had broken because of its age. You obtain a flat-plate abdominal study and note that the new peritoneal catheter is coiled neatly under the incision. What is the most likely diagnosis?**

Misplaced peritoneal shunt causing shunt malfunction.

○   **A 76 year old male is referred to you for evaluation of urinary incontinence. During the examination you note that he has trouble ambulating. Upon further questioning you find that he has had increasing gait difficulty for several months and admits to some memory loss. He has no back pain or other neurologic findings. His history is significant for a subarachnoid hemorrhage 15 years ago. CT scan of the head reveals ventriculomegaly out of proportion to brain atrophy. What is the most likely diagnosis?**

Normal pressure hydrocephalus (NPH).

○   *A multiple trauma patient is sleepy and confused after a transient loss of consciousness at the time of injury. The only external sign of injury is a seatbelt/shoulder strap bruise on the chest and neck. Initial head CT and neck x-rays are normal. The patient deteriorates over the next 12 hours from purposeful movement of all extremities to left hemiplegia. Repeat CT still reveals no obvious focal abnormalities. What is the most likely diagnosis?*

A missed injury of the right carotid artery.

○   **A 67 year old male is brought to the emergency room following a motor vehicle accident (MVA) of uncertain circumstances. Evaluation reveals a small basal ganglia hemorrhage that the radiologist describes as unusual for trauma. What is the most likely explanation for this patient's injuries?**

The patient most likely had a cerebral infarct that preceded the MVA.

○   **A child presents after falling from his bicycle. The parents, who were first on the scene, report that he appeared to be having a seizure. On examination he is now awake but drowsy. CT of the head is normal. The parents are obviously concerned after witnessing the seizure. What can you guardedly tell them about the child's prognosis for recovery and future seizures?**

Impact or immediate seizures can occur with traumatic incidents. However, they do not predispose the patient to future epilepsy.

○   **A multiple trauma patient is transferred to your facility with a history of head injury. The patient arrives intubated and sedated because he had a seizure prior to transport and was given 20 mg of intravenous diazepam. The patient now starts to seize again. The anesthesiologist offers to paralyze the patient. What is the appropriate treatment?**

Phenytoin.

○   **What complications can occur when anti-seizure medications are delivered too rapidly?**

Arrhythmias and hypotension.

○   **What is the role of lumbar puncture in the treatment of increased ICP?**

It is contraindicated. (It may lead to cerebellar or temporal herniation!)

○   **A trauma patient is found to have a significant acute subdural hematoma by CT scan. What is the appropriate treatment?**

Emergency craniotomy.

○   **What are the CT signs of diffuse, severe brain edema that are often associated with a dismal prognosis?**

Intracranial hypertension, cerebral herniation, loss of basal cisterns, compression of the ventricles and obliteration of the third ventricle.

○   **A 24 year old female presents with lethargy, dizziness, headache, nausea and vomiting. She has no medical problems other than chronic neck and back pain, for which she receives chiropractic manipulations. Her current symptoms started not long after a session with the chiropractor earlier that day. A CT of the head demonstrates hypodensity of the left cerebellum with associated edema. The radiologist wonders why such a healthy young patient would suffer from a posterior fossa region infarct. What is the possible physiology of the infarction?**

Atherosclerosis and hypertension are the main causes for posterior fossa infarcts.   However, any trauma to the vertebral arteries can manifest in a similar way. The vertebral arteries are vulnerable to blunt injury and significant cervical movements (i.e., MVAs, falls and manipulative therapies).

O   **What is the appropriate treatment for the above patient?**

Emergent posterior fossa decompression.

O   **A 35 year old female presents with a right hemisphere TIA. Evaluation reveals angiographic narrowing of the right internal carotid artery. The radiologist describes the appearance as a string of beads. What is the treatment of choice?**

Endovascular treatments, such as balloon angiography and intra-arterial stenting, may prove to be beneficial for fibromuscular dysplasia.

O   *A 70 year old male presents with acute right sided hemiparesis and mild aphasia that has improved since arrival to the emergency room. Angiography reveals complete occlusion of the left internal carotid artery. What is the appropriate management?*

Surgical intervention should be delayed for days to weeks since the symptoms are resolving. Furthermore, complete occlusion is not usually amenable to surgical intervention unless it is a hyperacute event.

O   **What is the role of surgery and adjunctive therapy in GBM?**

Patients receiving combined surgery and radiation therapies have a survival of 12 to 18 months.

O   **What is the mean survival for patients with untreated GBM?**

3 months.

O   **What is a type II odontoid fracture?**

A fracture between the dens and the body of C2 (at the synchondrosis). It is considered unstable and usually requires surgical intervention due to its poor vascular supply.

O   **What are the limitations of using stereotactic localization for brain lesions?**

Vascular compromise, sampling error and no reduction in mass.

O   *What is the origin of the artery of Adamkiewicz?*

It usually arises as a radicular artery from the descending aorta between T8 and L4.

O   **A patient presents with foot drop and back pain. What is the diagnostic test of choice?**

MRI. However, CT myelography can be used as an alternative or adjunctive study.

O   **What disc level most likely herniated in the above patient?**

L4-5.

O   *What is the most common neurosurgical problem in the pediatric age group?*

Trauma.

O   **How is a far-lateral lumbar disc herniation different from a central disc herniation?**

A far-lateral disc herniation implies that the herniated material is more on the posterolateral aspect of the disc space, within the lateral foramen.

○ **A 39 year old male presents to the emergency room after shoveling snow and complains of acute onset of severe low back pain. Evaluation reveals bilateral weakness of the feet on dorsiflexion, loss of sensation on the inner thighs and perineal regions and a distended bladder. What is the most likely diagnosis?**

Cauda equina syndrome.

○ **What is the appropriate treatment for the above patient?**

 Emergent surgical decompression with removal of the disc fragment(s).

○ **T/F: The presence of a pacemaker is a contraindication to MRI scanning.**

True.

○ **What diagnostic modality is indicated for the evaluation of the posterior fossa?**

MRI.

○ **A 74 year old woman with apathy, lethargy, expressive aphasia and left gaze deviation is likely to have what diagnosis?**
A glioblastoma of the left frontal lobe.

○ **What is the most common primary brain tumor?**

An astrocytoma.

○ *A patient who has coarse facial features and continues to increase shoe and glove size in adulthood has what type of tumor?*

A growth hormone-secreting pituitary adenoma.

○ *An obese woman with hypertension, diabetes and a large deposit of fat over the lower cervical and upper thoracic spine most likely has what diagnosis?*

Cushing's syndrome.

○ *A 53 year old female presents with spontaneous breast secretions and bitemporal field cuts. What is the most likely diagnosis?*

A prolactin secreting macroadenoma.

○ *Unilateral hearing loss and ipsilateral facial weakness are commonly seen with what tumor?*

An acoustic neuroma.

○ **What is the etiology of hyponatremia commonly seen after subarachnoid hemorrhage?**

Cerebral salt wasting due to excess atrial natriuretic factor.

○ **What is the most common cause of subarachnoid hemorrhage?**

Cerebral aneurysms.

❍ **What is the likelihood of rupture of an incidentally discovered intracranial aneurysm?**

1 to 3% per year.

❍ **What is the etiology of vasospasm following subarachnoid hemorrhage?**

Contraction of the smooth muscle cells in the cerebral vasculature secondary to breakdown of red blood cells and release of hemoglobin into the CSF.

❍ **A 50 year old woman presents with a complaint of hearing her pulse at night. Evaluation reveals a normal exam with no audible bruits. What is the most likely diagnosis?**

A dural arteriovenous malformation.

❍ **What is the appropriate treatment for an intracranial arteriovenous malformation?**

Surgical resection is the gold standard. However, newer therapies, including embolization, filling the malformation with glue or particulate matter and radiosurgery are being investigated.

❍ **What is the most likely cause of sudden painful exopthalmos with an ocular bruit?**

A carotid-cavernous fistula.

❍ *T/F: A patient with transient monocular blindness and a carotid bruit is best managed by carotid end-arterectomy (CEA).*

True.

❍ *How much does CEA decrease the risk of stroke in the asymptomatic population with stenosis > 50%?*

Up to 50%.

❍ **What is the best prophylactic treatment for CVA in patients with atrial fibrillation?**

Warfarin.

❍ **What organisms are most commonly implicated in subdural empyemas?**

Staphylococcus and streptococcus.

❍ **What is the window of opportunity for intravenous tPA administration following CVA?**

3 hours, assuming no early edema or blood is seen on CT.

❍ **What percentage of trauma related deaths are due to head injury?**

50%.

❍ **What is the mechanism of diffuse axonal injury?**

Rotation of the brain within the skull secondary to sudden deceleration.

❍ *Subdural hematomas and retinal hemorrhages in infants are pathognomonic of what syndrome?*

Shaken baby syndrome.

❍ **A baby with a myelomeningocele is likely to have what other neurologic malformation?**

A Chiari malformation.

○   **A 6 year old male presents after a mild head injury with a severe headache, nausea and diminished level of consciousness. CT scan of the head is normal. What do you instruct the distraught parents?**

Young children are often observed to have increased intracranial pressure after a mild head injury. This is thought to be due to a transient loss of autoregulation of cerebral blood flow and the outcome is usually good.

○   *What is the goal CPP in patients with brain injury?*

Greater than 70 mm Hg.

○   **What is the expected 5-year survival for low-grade astrocytomas?**

60%.

○   **What is the earliest sign of central herniation?**

Decreased level of consciousness.

○   **What physical findings are indicative of a basilar skull fracture?**

Periorbital ecchymosis, anterior fossa fractures (Battle's sign) and retromastoid ecchymosis with petrous fractures. Patients may also suffer hearing loss, anosmia and CSF leaks.

○   *What is the most common source of bleeding from an epidural hematoma?*

Laceration of the middle meningeal artery.

○   **What type of paralysis is expected from slow onset of spinal cord compression?**

Spastic paralysis.

○   *What is the source of bleeding from a subdural hematoma?*

Shearing of bridging veins between the dura and brain.

○   **What are clinical features of back pain secondary to tumors?**

Pain at night or unrelieved by recumbency.

○   *What reflex is affected by an L5-S1 herniated disc?*

The ankle jerk.

○   **A patient with normal reflexes, diminished grip strength and numbness over the 4th and 5th digits can be expected to have a herniated disc at what level?**

C7-T1.

○   **What are the advantages of the posterior approach for treatment of a herniated cervical disc?**

It avoids the structures of the anterior neck (i.e., the esophagus, carotid artery, jugular vein, vagus nerve and recurrent laryngeal nerves).

○   **What procedure is available for CSF diversion in young children with aqueductal stenosis?**

Endoscopic fenestration of the third ventricle.

○   **What are the most common symptoms of shunt malfunction in young children?**

Lethargy, irritability and, in advanced cases, forced downward gaze.

○   **What type of odontoid fracture is most likely to result in non-union with conservative therapy?**

Type II.

○   *What is the most common cause of a chance fracture?*

A high lap belt worn during an MVA.

○   **What is the most common type of astrocytoma?**

Malignant GBM.

GENITOURINARY PEARLS

The mind has great influence over the body, and maladies often have their origin there.

Molière

○ **What is the incidence of bladder and ureteral injuries in gynecological procedures and cesarean deliveries?**

1%.

○ **What is the most common gynecologic procedure associated with ureteral injury?**

Abdominal hysterectomy.

○ **What is the ratio of bladder injury to ureteral injury?**

5:1.

○ **What surgical factors are associated with ureteral or bladder injury?**

Misplaced sutures, difficult dissection and devascularization.

○ **What are the most common obstetrical factors associated with injury to the genitourinary tract?**

Forceps deliveries with trauma to the periurethral, anterior vaginal or lateral pelvic regions.

○ **What clinical conditions are associated with a higher risk of genitourinary injury?**

A large pelvic mass, pregnant uterus, obesity, pelvic hemorrhage, malignant disease and inadequate incision, traction and lighting.

○ **At what anatomical sites do ureteral injuries most often occur?**

Near the pelvic brim, at the infundibulopelvic ligament, at the base of the broad ligament where the ureter crosses the uterine artery and at the ureterovesical junction where the ureter moves medially to insert into the bladder.

○ **What is the best technique for dissecting the bladder away from the uterus in cases complicated by dense adhesive disease?**

Sharp dissection with retrograde filling of the bladder.

○ **What is the significance of spillage of indigo carmine into the pelvis?**

It is suggestive of urinary tract compromise.

○ **How do patients with ureteral obstruction present postoperatively?**

With flank pain, fever and leukocytosis.

○ **What effect does ureteral obstruction have on serum creatinine levels?**

It may be normal or slightly elevated.

○   **If urinary leakage is suspected, what tests on the recovered fluid are diagnostic?**

Measurement of creatinine or BUN will reveal levels many times greater than serum levels if urine is present.

○   **How are suspected urethral injuries identified?**

By urethroscopy or by placing a transurethral catheter.

○   **What are the treatment options for ureteral injuries discovered postoperatively?**

Immediate re-exploration and repair, immediate cystoscopic or percutaneous stenting of the damaged ureter.

○   **How can areas of ureteral stenosis be treated?**

Percutaneous placement of balloon stents or laparoscopic/surgical correction.

○   **T/F: Urinary sepsis is a contraindication to percutaneous stenting.**

False.

○   **What are the advantages of percutaneous or cystoscopic management of ureteral injuries?**

Correction can be done without general anesthesia, minimal morbidity and it decreases recovery time from laparotomy.

○   **What surgical techniques are available for treating ureteral injuries?**

Ureteroureterostomy, ureteroneocystostomy and transureteroureterostomy.

○   **What surgical techniques are available for treating urethral injuries?**

Removal of misplaced sutures and repair of lacerations in layers can be used to treat urethral injuries. Proximal urethral incontinence may require anterior colporaphy or bladder neck suspension.

○   **During hysterectomy, when do most ureteral injuries occur?**

During clamping the uterine vessels or ligation of the infundibulopelvic ligaments.

○   *T/F: Pts with Cryptorchidism are at 3-14x risk of testicular Ca this is a reason to operate?*

False. Operation does not decrease cancer risk, only increases fertility.

○   *PT present with a varicocele of the left testicle what should you be concerned about?*

Retroperitoneal or renal mass because the left gonadal vein drains into the L renal vein.

○   **T/F: Bladder injury encountered during a vaginal hysterectomy is an indication to abort the procedure.**

False.

○   **Where do most bladder injuries associated with laparoscopic surgery occur?**

The dome of the bladder.

○ *Which laparoscopic bladder injuries can be managed conservatively?*

Punctures involving 5 to 7 mm trocars will self-seal with prolonged transurethral drainage. Similarly, small caliber bladder injury caused by cautery or lasers may be treated with prolonged drainage.

○ **What surgical procedures most commonly result in vesicovaginal fistulas?**

Total abdominal or vaginal hysterectomy.

○ **How does management of ureteral injuries differ during a radical hysterectomy, as opposed to a non-radical procedure?**

The extensive ureteral dissection compromises ureteral blood supply, so reimplantation of the ureter is preferential to attempts at reanastomosis or closure of ureteral injuries.

○ *How should a partially transected ureter be managed?*

With several interrupted sutures, stenting and retroperitoneal drainage.

○ *A trauma pt has blood at urethral meatus and a high riding prostate, what test do you order?*

Retrograde urethragram, before you place a foley; if urethral disruption has occurred, supra-pubic cystostomy should be placed.

○ *What are the treatments for extra peritoneal and intraperitoneal bladder rupture?*

Extra peritoneal- foley.
Intraperitoneal- foley and multi- layer bladder closure in OR.

○ **What factors determine the type of procedure appropriate for repair of a totally transected ureter?**

Level of the ureteral transection, length of the damaged segment, mobility of the ureter/bladder, quality of the pelvic tissue, the underlying indication for the procedure and the general health and expected lifetime of the patient.

○ *How are injuries to the pelvic ureter best treated?*

By ureteroneocystotomy.

○ **How do the left and right ureters differ in their pelvic course?**

The left ureter enters the pelvis and crosses the common iliac artery more medially than the right.

○ **How is ureteral obstruction due to endometriosis best managed?**

Resection.

○ **T/F: Preoperative stenting decreases the risk of ureteral injury.**

False.

○ **What problems are associated with preoperative ureteral stenting?**

Colicky pain, hematuria and ureteral fibrosis.

○ **During a hysterectomy, what does reflecting the bladder inferiorly due to the position of the ureter?**

It displaces the ureter laterally, making uterine artery division safer.

○   **If ureteral injury is recognized during a hysterectomy, when should it be repaired?**

After the uterus is removed.

○   **How does pelvic irradiation affect the ureter?**

The blood supply is compromised, the ureter appears more pale and is harder to palpate, connective tissue of the broad ligament is more difficult to dissect from the ureter and, rarely, obstruction may result.

○   **If ureteral obstruction is detected in a patient after radiation for cancer of the cervix, what is the most likely cause?**

Recurrent tumor.

○   **During dissection, how is the ureter best handled?**

Carefully and gently with a wet Penrose drain, umbilical tape or fine tipped non-toothed forceps. Traction is best given by pulling on tissue next to the ureter, not by pulling on the ureter.

○   **What type of suture is best for bladder or ureteral repairs?**

Fine caliber absorbable suture.

○   **T/F: We operate on Cryptorchidism so that the young man can look normal in the locker room.**

False. The testicle have faulty sperm production when the testicle has elevated temp, as occurs when undescended. Thus fertility is increased s/p operation. Operate after 1 year if not descended on own.

○   *What is the initial clinical effect of acute tubular necrosis (ATN) on renal function?*

Loss of urinary concentrating ability.

○   **What level of spinal or epidural blockade is required to suppress the sympathetic response to hypotension and surgical stress and maintain renal blood flow?**

T4 to T10.

○   **What is the mechanism of renal toxicity due to volatile anesthetic agents?**

The production of free fluoride ions.

○   *What is the effect of PEEP on renal function?*

It can decrease cardiac output and, thus, renal blood flow, glomerular filtration rate and urine output.

○   **What is the effect of trimethophan on renal blood flow?**

It abolishes autoregulation and decreases renal vascular resistance.

○   *What factors predispose to renal failure in myoglobinemia secondary to rhabdomyolysis?*

Low urine pH (less than 5.6) and hypovolemia.

○   **How does urine specific gravity and osmolality help determine renal tubular function?**

A high specific gravity (greater than 1.030) or a high osmolality (greater than 1050 mOsm/kg) implies unimpaired tubular function. Urine specific gravity (1.010) or osmolality (290 mOsm/kg) that is the same as plasma is suggestive of renal disease. A dilute urine (50-100 mOsm/kg) may still indicate renal disease, as the urine dilution mechanism fails after the concentrating ability.

O   *Why is a normal serum creatinine still consistent with impaired renal function, especially in the elderly?*

Serum creatinine concentrations are dependent on dietary protein intake and muscle tissue turnover. Elderly people have less muscle mass and, thus, lower serum creatinines.

O   **How does chronic renal failure (CRF) affect protein binding?**

It decreases it by 10%.

O   **Why should pancuronium be used cautiously in patients with renal failure?**

Pancuronium is 40 to 50% excreted in the urine and one of the hepatic metabolites (3-hyrodoxypancuronium) is active and excreted in the urine.

O   **A CRF patient who requires regular hemodialysis develops weakness and mild respiratory distress in the post-anesthetic care unit. The patient received vecuronium, which was reversed at the end of the procedure with neostigmine and atropine. What is the most likely explanation?**

Interaction between an antibiotic, diuretic or electrolyte disturbance with the muscle relaxant.

O   *What are the problems with the use of sodium nitroprusside in patients with renal impairment?*

The half-life of thiocyanate, one of the metabolites is prolonged. This may result in hypoxia, nausea, tinnitus, muscle spasm and/or psychosis if levels exceed 10 mg/100 ml. With prolonged elevation, hypothyroidism may result.

O   **What determines the absorption of irrigating solutions during transurethral resection of the prostate?**

The height of the irrigating solution above the patient (hydrostatic pressure) and the duration of surgery.

O   **What level of spinal anesthesia is desirable for a TURP?**

T10.

O   **What are the absolute contraindications to extracorporeal shock wave lithotripsy (ESWL)?**

Pregnancy and bleeding disorders.

O   **What degree of nephron loss and fall in creatinine clearance is associated with uremia?**

Loss of 95% of functioning nephrons and a fall in creatinine clearance to less than 12 ml/minute.

O   *What is the fractional excretion of sodium (FeNa)?*

(Urinary sodium/plasma sodium) divided by (urinary creatinine/plasma creatinine) x 100.

O   **What level of regional anesthesia is required for ESWL?**

A block up to the T6 level.

○   **What is the importance of ECG monitoring during ESWL?**

There is a risk of cardiac dysrhythmias due to the discharge of shock waves independent of the cardiac cycle.

○   **For patients undergoing a renal transplant, when would preoperative blood transfusion be appropriate?**

If the hemoglobin is lower than the patients usual chronically low level (often 6-8g/dl) or if the transplant team feels that the use of a blood transfusion may enhance allograft survival.

○   **T/F: Succinylcholine is a safe choice in the renal failure patient.**

True. If the patient has been recently dialyzed and the potassium is normal, succinylcholine is an appropriate choice, if indicated.

○   **What hemodynamic variables must to be considered in a patient recently dialyzed who is about to undergo anesthesia?**

Following dialysis, patients are usually hypovolemic. They also often take antihypertensive medication as well as the possible hypotensive interaction with various anesthetic agents.

○   **What are the potential side effects of cyclosporin (an immunosuppressive agent often used in renal transplant patients)?**

Renal and hepatic toxicity, hypertension, hyperuricemia and seizures.

○   **What is the average absorption rate of irrigation fluid during a TURP?**

Between 10 and 30 ml/minute.

○   **What is the most common cause of painless hematuria in children?**

A glomerular lesion.

○   *What is the function of atrial natriuretic peptide (ANP)?*

It relaxes vascular smooth muscle, decreases sympathetic stimulation and inhibits renin and aldosterone secretion.

○   **Why may the use of NSAIDs be a concern in patients with hypovolemia or renal impairment?**

Blockade of prostaglandin-mediated effects on renal blood flow by NSAIDs predisposes these patients to developing renal failure.

○   **What are the most common causes of urinary urgency?**

Prostatitis, urethritis or cystitis.

○   *What is the most common cause of acute left varicocele?*

Renal vein occlusion (commonly related to renal tumors).

○   *When a patient presents to the emergency room with sudden onset of severe testicular pain, what is the most likely diagnosis and why is it important to make the diagnosis quickly?*

Testicular torsion. If the torsion is not corrected within 4 hours, there may be irreversible damage to the testis.

❍ **What types of kidney stones are associated with perinephric abscesses?**

Struvite or staghorn calculi.

❍ **What is the most common manifestation of metastatic gonococcal infection?**

Gonococcal arthritis (80%).

❍ **What is the most common venereal disease in males?**

Nonspecific urethritis.

❍ **What is the etiology of urinary tuberculosis?**

Hematogenous spread from primary pulmonary or intestinal lesions.

❍ **What type of kidney stone is associated with primary hyperparathyroidism?**

Hydroxyapatite crystal predominance.

❍ **What percentage of urinary tract stones are radiopaque?**

90%.

❍ **When is ESWL most effective in the treatment of urinary tract stones?**

When the stones are less than 2 cm in size.

❍ **What is the primary defect of absorptive hypercalciuria?**

Intestinal hyperabsorption of calcium.

❍ **What is the most common site of adenocarcinoma of the prostate?**

The peripheral zone.

❍ **What are the best tests for detecting prostate cancer?**

Digital rectal exam and measurement of serum prostatic specific antigen (PSA).

❍ **What is the mechanism of action of alpha-blockers in the treatment of BPH?**

It relaxes the smooth muscle and partially relieves the dynamic component of obstruction.

❍ **What is the most common cancer affecting the kidney?**

Renal cell carcinoma (85%).

❍ **What is the most common cancer affecting the kidney in childhood?**

Wilm's tumor (adenomyosarcoma).

❍ **What is the classical triad of clinical manifestations seen in patients with renal tumors?**

Pain, palpable mass and hematuria. However, they occur late and in only about 50% of patients.

❍ **What is the standard surgical procedure for unilateral renal neoplasms?**

Radical nephrectomy with removal of the ipsilateral adrenal and hilar nodes.

❍ **What is the overall survival rate for patients with renal carcinoma?**

70%.

❍ **On histological examination of a renal tumor, it is found to be mahogany-colored, well-demarcated and has a central area of necrosis. The cells have abundant granular eosinophilic cytoplasm. What is the most likely diagnosis?**

Oncocytoma.

❍ **A 49 year old white male with a history of tuberous sclerosis, seizures and mental retardation presents to the emergency room with systemic sepsis. A CT of the abdomen and pelvis reveal a solitary mass in the right kidney. What is the most likely diagnosis?**

Angiomyolipoma.

❍ **In what region of the kidney do hemangiomas most often occur?**

In the renal pelvis.

❍ **Which renal tumor shows renin granules on electromicroscopy and is a cause of secondary aldosteronism with severe hypertension?**

Juxtaglomerular tumors.

❍ **What is the most common tumor affecting the renal pelvocalyceal system?**

Transitional cell carcinoma.

❍ **What is the appropriate treatment for bladder stones?**

Cystoscopic removal and correction of predisposing factors.

❍ **A 55 year old male presents with gross hematuria and renal colic. IVP shows a filling defect in the left mid-ureter. What is the most likely diagnosis?**

Transitional cell carcinoma.

❍ **A 70 year old white male smoker with a history of prolonged exposure to beta-napthalene presents with microhematuria and dysuria. What is the most likely diagnosis?**

Transitional cell carcinoma of the bladder.

❍ **What percentage of prostatic nodules palpated by digital rectal exam are posit264ve for cancer on biopsy?**

50%.

❍ **What is the risk of a 50 year old male developing impotence following prostatectomy? A 70 year old?**

50 and 80%, respectively.

❍ **What therapeutic options are available for the patient with prostate cancer who cannot tolerate surgery or radiation?**

Estrogen therapy, androgen blockade or orchiectomy.

❍ **What is the most common testicular tumor?**

Seminoma (40%).

❍ **What is the relative incidence of testicular tumors in patients with an abdominal undescended testicle?**

50 times greater than the normal population. (The risk does not change even if the testicle is brought down to its normal location.)

❍ **Which testicular tumor in most common in older men?**

Seminoma.

❍ *What is the preferred surgical approach to a lesion confined to the testis on physical exam?*

The inguinal approach.

❍ **What must be done prior to exteriorization of the testis to prevent spread of tumor?**

Occlusion of the spermatic vessels.

❍ **If, during exploration for a testicular tumor, the testis is found to be indurated, what procedure should be performed?**

Radical orchiectomy.

❍ **What are the indications for retroperitoneal nodal dissection in a patient with a testicular tumor?**

CT-defined nodal involvement, invasion of lymphatics or blood vessels within the parenchyma by nonseminomatous tumors, persistence of a large volume of teratocarcinoma within the testis and failure of markers to return to normal after removal of a testicle containing nonseminomatous germ cell elements.

❍ **What is the recommended postoperative adjuvant therapy for Stage A seminomas?**

27 to 36 cGy to the abdomen.

❍ **What is the postoperative adjuvant treatment for Stage C seminoma?**

Chemotherapy alone.

❍ **What is the treatment for Stage B and C embryonal cell tumors?**

Chemotherapy alone or followed by retroperitoneal lymph node dissection.

❍ *Which testicular tumor has the best 5-year survival?*

Seminoma.

❍ **Which testicular tumor has the worst prognosis?**

Choriocarcinoma (it is almost always fatal).

❍ **Which testicular tumor is the most radiosensitive?**

Seminoma.

O   **How does priapism differ from a true erection?**

With priapism, the glans and the bulbospongiosus are not erect but the corpora cavernosa are.

O   **What is the treatment for priapism?**

Slow injection of a few millimeters of 1:100,000 epinephrine directly into the corpora.

O   **What is the sperm count in a normal healthy male?**
Between 30 and 100 million sperm/ml with at least 70% showing purposeful motility.

O   **What is the most likely diagnosis if the ejaculate lacks fructose?**

A ductal obstruction.

O   **In what percentage of patients who have suffered blunt trauma to the kidney is hematuria absent?**

20%.

O   **What grade(s) of renal injuries can usually be managed nonoperatively?**

Grades 1, 2 and 3. They are treated with bed rest until hematuria resolves.

O   **What are the indications for surgery in a patient who has sustained traumatic renal injury?**

Urinary extravasation, persistent retroperitoneal bleeding and nonviable tissue.

O   **What is the best surgical approach for renal exploration after trauma?**

Midline abdominal.

O   **What is the most common cause of ureteral injury?**

Iatrogenic injury during abdominal procedures.

O   **A patient returns for follow-up after sustaining a rapid deceleration motor vehicle accident two weeks prior. He complains of flank pain, has a palpable mass and shows ileus on abdominal films. What is the most likely GU associated diagnosis?**

A missed ureteral injury with development of a urinoma.

O   *What is the treatment of choice for injuries to the middle or upper third of the ureter?*

Primary ureteroureterostomy over a J stent.

O   **What percentage of bladder injuries are extraperitoneal?**

75%.

O   *What is the most common cause of traumatic bladder injury?*

Pelvic fracture with penetration of the bladder by bone spicules.

O   **What percentage of pelvic fractures have an associated bladder or urethral injury?**

5 to 15%.

○   *What is the treatment for most extraperitoneal bladder injuries?*

Conservative management with catheter drainage.

○   *What is the treatment of choice for an intraperitoneal bladder injury?*

A 2-layer closure with suprapubic drainage for several weeks.

○   *What is the most common cause of urethral injury?*

Pelvic fracture or perineal penetration (saddle injury).

○   *What is the initial procedure for patients with documented urethral injury?*

Cystostomy.

○   **What is the typical presentation of a urethral valve anomaly?**

A young boy with a weak or dribbling stream.

○   **What are the possible complications of an unrepaired urethral valve anomaly?**

Uremia and hypertension.

○   **What is the treatment for urethral valve anomalies?**

Destruction of the valves.

○   **How is the diagnosis of neurogenic bladder confirmed?**

Excretory urography, voiding cystourethogram and cystometry. A positive finding includes large residual urine with low-pressure, high-volume tracings and lack of sensation of filling until large volumes have been instilled.

○   **What is the characteristic complaint of women with an ectopic ureteral orifice?**

Urinary incontinence despite normal voiding habits.

○   **What congetinal anomaly is associated with infantile or ectopic ureterocele?**

Duplication of the drainage system.

○   **What is the typical appearance on IVP that indicates a ureterocele?**

A cobra-head deformity.

○   **What conditions are associated with vesicoureteral reflux (VUR)?**

Posterior urethral valves, prune-belly syndrome, complete duplication of the collecting system, Ask-Upmark kidney (segmental renal hypoplasia), neurogenic bladder, bladder neck obstruction, tuberculosis, bladder infections, suprapubic and indwelling urethral catheters and bladder-urethral dysynergia.

○   **What is required to conclude disappearance of reflux?**

Two consecutive normal VCUGs at least 12 months apart.

○   **In what condition is the most severely dilated urinary tracts found?**

Prune-belly syndrome.

○   **What is the pathologic cause of uretopelvic obstruction?**

Deficiency of longitudinal muscle at the ureteropelvic junction.

○   **What is the usual outcome for patients with adult polycystic kidney disease?**

Renal failure.

○   **What percentage of premature males have undescended testicle? Full-term males?**

30% and 4%, respectively.

○   **What is the critical finding that must be ruled out when a varicocele is detected?**

A retroperitoneal tumor.

○   **What are the indications for repair of a varicocele?**

Size, scrotal pain, rapid growth and subfertility with abnormal sperm in the ejaculate.

○   *A 2 year old male is brought to the emergency room by his mother who states that his scrotum is enlarged during the day but decreases in size at night. What is the most likely diagnosis?*

A hydrocele.

○   **What is the most common form of the adrenogenital syndrome (CAH)?**

46, XX/21-hydroxylase variant (90%).

○   **What is the most common fusion defect of the urethra?**

Hypospadias (1:300 male births).

○   **What is the most common location of the urethral meatus in a patient with hypospadias?**

At the distal end of the penile shaft, anteriorly.

○   **What are the indications for a lumbar approach in performing a nephrectomy?**

Inflammatory renal disease, calculi, perinephric abscess, hydronephrosis and renal cystic disease.

○   **What are the indications for performing a cutaneous ureteroileostomy (ileal conduit)?**

Removal or the urinary bladder and impaired bladder detrusor function.

PEDIATRIC SURGERY PEARLS

Adults are obsolete children —— and the hell with them.
Theodore Geisel (Dr. Seuss)

O   **How does an omphalocele usually present?**

As a mass of bowel and solid viscera in the central abdomen, covered by a translucent membrane.

O   **What are the indications for nonoperative treatment of an omphalocele?**

Presence of other life-threatening anomalies, whose corrections takes precedence and patients with other anomalies that may not be consistent with life.

O   **Why is the prognosis for gastroschisis worse than that for an omphalocele?**

Because of the amount of time the abdominal contents is spent being bathed in irritating amniotic fluid.

O   **When should primary closure be attempted in a patient with gastroschisis?**

When the intragastric pressure is less than 20 cm H2O and the central venous pressure (CVP) does not increase by 4 mm Hg or more as the abdominal viscera are replaced into the abdominal cavity.

O   **If primary closure can not be performed, how is the abdominal wall closed?**

Usually with a silastic sheet fashioned into a chimney or silo, the volume of which can be decreased day-to-day. Once the height of the silo is level with the rest of the abdominal wall, the infant is returned to the operating room for surgical abdominal wall closure.

O   **What is the etiology of a congenital diaphragmatic hernia?**

Typically, the abdominal viscera herniate through a defect in the central tendon of the left hemidiaphragm into the left hemithorax.

O   **What classic triad is seen in patients with a congenital diaphragmatic hernia?**

Respiratory distress, cyanosis and apparent dextrocardia.

O   **What is the mortality of congenital diaphragmatic hernia?**

50%.

O   **What are the major goals of perioperative management for neonates severely affected by a congenital diaphragmatic hernia?**

To prevent occurrence of hypoxemia and acidosis by maximizing ventilation and oxygenation and by minimizing metabolic stressors.

O   **How will the pathophysiology typically evolve if the above goals cannot be met?**

1.   Hypoxemia and acidosis induce pulmonary vasoconstriction.

2. Increased pulmonary vascular resistance produces an elevation in right ventricular and right atrial pressures, as well as pulmonary artery pressures.
3. Elevated right-sided perfusion pressures and resistances induce a return to the fetal circulatory state, with reopening of the foramen ovale and ductus arteriosus.
4. This persistent fetal circulation induces further hypoxemia and acidosis, eventually resulting in multiple organ failure and death.

O   **What other congenital anomalies are often seen with congenital diaphragmatic hernia?**

Other midline defects, including congenital heart disease (i.e., patent ductus arteriosus).

O   **What bowel segments are typically involved in intestinal atresias?**

The duodenum, jejunum, terminal ileum and anus.

O   **What non-invasive diagnostic test can reliably contribute to the decision making process in pyloric stenosis?**

Ultrasound.

O   **Infants with pyloric stenosis, whose diagnosis was delayed, may present with what metabolic disturbances?**

Dehydration, hypochloremic metabolic alkalosis and hypokalemia.

O   **What is the leading cause of death in childhood?**

Trauma.

O   **T/F: Pyloric stenosis is a surgical emergency.**

False.

O   *What is the most common type of choledochal cyst?*

Type I, involves the CBD only, treatement is hepatico-jejunostomy.

O   *In Pulmonary Sequestration What type of circulation is associated with Extra lobar and Intra lobar?*

Extra lobar- systemic artery and veins.
Intralobar- systemic inflow and pulmonary vein outflow.

O   **How does a patient most commonly present with pulmonary sequestration?**

Infection.

O   **What is the most common complication of cystic hygroma and what is the treatment?**

Infection   Tx: Resection.

O   **If a patient with a tracheo-esophageal fistula, of the proximal esophageal pouch variety, also has congenital heart disease, how should the various surgeries be planned?**

Attention should first be turned to the fistula. Once the risk to the lungs has been minimized, consideration can be given to the congenital heart disease. Unless the patient has cyanotic heart disease, immediate reparative or palliative surgery of the heart and great vessels is usually not necessary.

○   **What problems do children with a history of tracheo-esophageal fistula repair encounter as they grow?**

They typically have reactive airway disease or other lung disease suggestive of chronic aspiration. They may also experience esophageal stenosis at the anastomotic site and require repeated bougienage and dilatation.

○   **T/F: Most airway foreign bodies are radio-opaque.**

False. As a rule, airway foreign bodies are radiolucent.

○   **How is the diagnosis of airway foreign body made?**

History of choking or coughing during play or eating, persistent cough, fever, infiltrate on chest x-ray and persistent high lung volume on decubitus x-ray suggesting air trapping.

○   **What is the special risk of peanut extraction from the airway?**

The peanut may shatter, causing particles to be spread to both lungs.

○   **Why does a patient not improve immediately after airway foreign body extraction?**

It takes time for the inflammatory response to dissipate.

○   **What is the preferred maintenance fluid for children older than 6 months of age?**

5% dextrose in 0.45% saline.

○   **For younger infants?**

5% dextrose in 0.2% saline. (The immature kidney is less able to handle a solute load.)

○   **What is the preferred crystalloid for replacement of extracellular fluid or third space losses?**

Lactated Ringer's, normal saline or other similar fluid.

○   **How do platelet transfusions affect the peripheral blood platelet count?**

A 10 ml/kg transfusion will increase the platelet count by ~150,000/mm^3. Each unit of platelets has ~50 ml volume. Thus, 1 unit per 5 kg will raise the platelet count by 150,000/mm^3.

○   **A 3 year old is scheduled for tonsillectomy. He has a runny nose, is coughing and sneezing but has no other symptoms. His 6 year old brother has had a cold for the past week. Mom says that he is always like this. How would you proceed?**

It is not likely that this child is at increased risk for perioperative anesthetic complications secondary to an upper respiratory infection. The operation can go ahead as planned.

○   **How is croup clinically differentiated from epiglottitis?**

Croup is most prevalent in infants, whereas epiglottitis is more prevalent in toddlers and pre-schoolers. Epiglottitis is associated with high fevers, toxic appearance and a brief course before the onset of respiratory distress. Croup, however, is usually more subacute in onset with a lower temperature and WBC count.

○   **A cyst like structure is found in neck of infant which is midline and moves with swallowing. What is the treatment for this abnormality?**

Excision of the Throglossal duct cyst with the hyoid bone.

○   *What is the treatment of Strawberry Hemangioma?*
Nothing. Most resolve by age 7.

○   **Which Tumor of childhood is the most common malignancy in child, and is associated with increased VMA and associated with N-myc?**

Neuroblastoma.

○   **What is the Rule of 2's for Meckel's diverticulum?**

2 ft from IC valve.
2% population.
2% symptomatic.
2 types of tissue: pancreas and gastric.
2 presentations: Gi bleed and diverticulitis.

○   **What is the immediate treatment for patients with epiglottitis?**

Direct laryngoscopy followed by tracheal intubation under general anesthesia in the operating room.

○   **What is the initial fluid resuscitation in a pediatric patient with hypotension?**

A 20 cc/kg normal saline bolus. This should be followed by a second bolus if an inadequate response is obtained. Consideration should be given to the use of blood if no response is noted after the second bolus.

○   **What are the most common organisms encountered in cervical lymphadenitis?**

Group A streptococcus and Staphylococcus aureus.

○   *What is the most common type of tracheo-esophageal fistula?*

A blind-ending proximal esophageal pouch with a fistula from the lower esophagus to the trachea (85%).

○   **What percentage of children less than 5 years of age will have a perforated appendicitis at the time of initial presentation?**

More than 50%.

○   **What is a normal urine output for a newborn baby?**

1 to 2 cc/kg/hour.

○   **What is the incidence of a contralateral inguinal hernia in an infant who presents with a unilateral hernia?**

50% or more.

○   **What are the fundamental steps required in a Ladd procedure?**

Detorsion of a volvulus, if present, division of Ladd's bands overlying the duodenum, mobilization and straightening of the duodenum and appendectomy.

○   **T/F: Passage of meconium excludes the diagnosis of jejunoileal atresia.**

False.

○   **What is the estimated blood volume of a child?**

80 cc/kg.

O   **What is the differential diagnosis for a midline neck mass in a child?**

Thyroglossal duct cyst, dermoid cyst or adenopathy.

O   **What is the most common branchial cleft anomaly?**

A second branchial cleft sinus.

O   **What is the anatomic location of most congenitally acquired diaphragmatic hernias?**

More than 80% occur in the left posterolateral chest through the foramen of Bochdalek.

O   *What are the anatomic features characteristic of pulmonary sequestration?*

A systemic blood supply (frequently subdiaphragmatic) and an absence of communication with the tracheobronchial tree.

O   **What associated anomalies must be excluded in the evaluation of the neonate with esophageal atresia?**

Those of the VATER or VACTERRL syndrome (Vertebral, Anorectal, Cardiac, Tracheo-Esophageal, Radial, Renal and Limb).

O   **What genetic abnormality may be present in up to 30% of newborns with duodenal atresia?**

Trisomy 21 (Down's syndrome).

O   **What is the preferred treatment for duodenal atresia?**

Duodenoduodenostomy.

O   **What is the etiology of a cystic hygroma (congenital lymphangiomatous malformation)?**

Sequestration or obstruction of developing lymph vessels.

O   **What are the most common locations for a cystic hygroma?**

The posterior triangle of the neck, axilla, groin and mediastinum (anywhere lymphatics are prominent). Cystic Hygroma=lymphangioma.

O   **What is the most common cause of colonic obstruction in infants?**

Hirschsprung's disease.

O   *What is the gold standard for the diagnosis of Hirschsprung's in the newborn period?*

The absence of ganglion cells in the submucosal and myenteric plexuses on rectal biopsy.

O   **In the child with recurrent urinary tract infections and persistent clear drainage from the umbilicus, what diagnosis should be considered and what study is most likely to demonstrate the problem?**

A patent urachus should be suspected and is best investigated with a contrast cystogram.

❍   *What is the inheritance pattern of familial adenomatous polyposis? At what age are polyps generally present?*

Familial adenomatous polyposis is transmitted as an autosomal dominant syndrome with high penetrance. Polyps are present in 15% of children by age 10 and over 98% by age 30.

❍   *A contrast enema is used in the evaluation of possible intussusception. How often is this method effective at reduction and what is the risk of recurrence following enema reduction?*

A contrast (air, barium or water-soluble) enema will successfully reduce an intussusception in 80% of cases. Recurrence is seen in 10 to 15% of patients, most commonly in the first 24 hours following reduction.

❍   **What are the relative indications for operative intervention in necrotizing enterocolitis?**

Abdominal wall erythema, fixed abdominal mass, portal venous air or a persistently dilated bowel loop on abdominal radiograph.

❍   **What is the most common malignant childhood malignancy?**

Leukemia.

❍   **What are the generally accepted contraindications to the use of extracorporeal membrane oxygenation (ECMO) in the neonate?**

Weight less than 2 kg and gestational age less than 34 weeks are exclusion criteria because of risk for intracranial hemorrhage (89% incidence in this population). Other exclusion criteria include irreversible lung disease, severe chromosomal or cardiac abnormalities or uncontrolled coagulopathy.

❍   **What is the most common hepatic malignancy in a child less than 4 years old?**

Hepatoblastoma.

❍   **What is the most common hepatic malignancy in a child greater than 4 years old?**

Hepatocellular carcinoma.

❍   **What is the differential diagnosis of an anterior mediastinal mass in a child?**

Thymoma, teratoma, lymphoma, ectopic thyroid tissue, cystic hygroma or lipoma.

❍   **What is the most common soft tissue tumor of childhood?**

Rhabdomyosarcoma.

❍   **What is the embryologic remnant which causes a Meckel's diverticulum?**

Omphalomesenteric duct.

❍   **What is the diagnositic and therapeutic treatment of meconium ileus?**

Gastrograffin enema.

❍   **In intussusception what test should be done before the Barium enema?**

An abdominal x-ray looking for free air. As do not give contrast if free air., go directly to the OR.

❍   *What are intestinal atresias secondary to?*

Intra-uterine vascular occlusion.

O **What is the most common location for a rhabdomyosarcoma in the pediatric age group?**

The head and neck region.

O **Inadvertent violation of the mucosa occurs in approximately 1% of pyloromyotomies. What are the treatment options for such an occurrence?**

Repair of the mucosal defect and omental patch or roll the pylorus 45° and perform a second myotomy after repair of the initial site.

O **What is the incidence of incarceration of inguinal hernias in the pediatric patient?**

6 to 18% of uncorrected inguinal hernias. In infants less than 2 months of age, the risk of incarceration may be as high as 30%.

O **What is the differential diagnosis for a posterior mediastinal mass in a child?**

Bronchogenic cyst, esophageal duplication cyst, neuroblastoma, ganglioneuroma or pulmonary sequestration.

O **What is the preferred method of airway control in the injured child?**

Placement of an oral airway and bag mask ventilation should be the initial approach. If more secure airway control is necessary, orotracheal intubation should be obtained. If these measures fail or are not appropriate, needle cricothyroidotomy is the method of choice.

O **What is the role of surgery in a pediatric rhabdomyosarcomas?**

Surgical resection prior to chemotherapy is the ideal management if an acceptable cosmetic and functional result can be obtained. Re-excision of the tumor bed in the setting of positive margins prior to chemotherapy has also been shown to be of benefit.

O **A 3 week old male presents with jaundice and a conjugated hyperbilirubinemia. Viral serologies are negative. What is the surgical approach to exclude the diagnosis of biliary atresia?**

A limited exploratory laparotomy with intraoperative cholangiogram and liver biopsy is the standard approach. Failure to demonstrate extrahepatic biliary ductal patency necessitates hepatic portoenterostomy for biliary drainage. This procedure is most efficacious when performed prior to 8 weeks of life.

O **What is the most common cause of rectal bleeding in the child over 1 year of age?**

Juvenile polyps.

O **What is the major perioperative concern in a child undergoing biopsy of an anterior mediastinal mass?**

Tracheal compression.

O **What are the operative indications for patients with typhlitis, a necrotizing colitis localized to the cecum?**

Persistent gastrointestinal bleeding despite resolution of thrombocytopenia and neutropenia, free intraperitoneal air, clinical deterioration requiring vasopressor support and evidence of an intraabdominal process, such as an abscess.

O **What clinical variables determine prognosis for patients with a neuroblastoma?**

The age of the patient and the stage of the disease at time of diagnosis and the site of the primary tumor.

○   **An 8 year old male presents with profound hypothermia from a near drowning in icy waters. What are the treatment options to achieve active rewarming?**

Heated intravenous fluids, heated inspired respiratory gases, warmed gastric or colonic lavage, warmed peritoneal or pleural lavage, hemodialysis or ECMO.

○   **What is the appropriate management for a deep puncture wound from a dog or cat bite?**

Post-exposure rabies prophylaxis should be considered for all bites. If the animal is healthy, it should be quarantined for 10 days to exclude rabies. If the animal is unavailable or suspected rabid, immediate vaccination and immunoglobulin therapy should be administered. In addition, antibiotic coverage to include Pastuerella multocida, should be initiated.

○   **What is the most common location of a gonadal germ cell tumor in childhood?**

The ovary.

○   **What is the most common location of an extragonadal germ cell tumor in childhood?**

The saccrococcygeal region.

○   *What is the presumed diagnosis in a patient with bilious emesis until proven otherwise?*

Malrotation of the midgut.

○   **What is the operative management for a patient with malrotation of the midgut?**

Counterclockwise reduction of the volvulus, if present, and resection of nonviable bowel.

○   **What is the diagnostic algorithm for the patient above if he/she is unstable and is suspected of having a bowel obstruction?**

Exploratory laparotomy.

○   **A patient is referred for management of an incidentally discovered abdominal mass thought to be a duplication cyst. What is the most likely location of this cyst?**

Cystic duplications can be found in any segment of the gastrointestinal tract, however, they are most common in the small intestine, in particular near the terminal ileum.

○   **What is the role of surgery in the above patient?**

Surgical resection is indicated for all duplication cysts as the origin and natural history of these lesions is poorly understood.

○   **What is the initial surgical approach to the child with a large renal-based mass?**

The diagnosis of exclusion is a Wilm's tumor. After preoperative evaluation (abdominal and chest CT) exploration of the abdomen is undertaken to rule out metastatic disease.

○   **What is the incidence of bilateral disease in a patient with a Wilm's tumor?**

5%.

○   **What is the most common diagnosis leading to liver transplantation in the pediatric population?**

Biliary atresia.

O **What are the expected 1-, 5- and 10-year survival rates following liver transplantation in the pediatric age group?**

76%, 71% and 61%, respectively.

O *What is the most common indication for splenectomy during childhood?*

Hereditary spherocytosis.

O **What is the most common intraabdominal tumor diagnosed during childhood?**

Wilm's tumor.

O *What is the most common indication for cholecystectomy in the pediatric age group?*

Cholelithiasis secondary to sickle cell disease.

O *What is the goal of surgery in children with a choledochal cyst?*

Removal of the cyst to prevent the late development of malignancy and to establish adequate biliary drainage to prevent cholangitis (hepaticojejunostomy for type 1).

O *What is the treatment of choice for patients with biliary atresia?*

Hepatoportoenterostomy (Kasai procedure).

O **A 3 year old male presents with a firm neck mass. Examination reveals Horner's syndrome. What is the most likely diagnosis?**

Neuroblastoma.

O **What is the most common cause of cervical adenopathy in children?**

Inflammation.

O *Duodenal atresia are associated with what?*

Double bubble on contrast study.
Duodenal obstruction.
Down's.

O *What should one think of in a child who can't tolerate feeds and NGT will not pass?*

TEF.

O *What is the most Common type of TE fistula?*

Type C. Blind esophagus, no distal TEF.

O **A 4 month old female has had a progressive barking cough and inspiratory stridor for 2 months. Examination reveals a raised, bright red lesion on her back that has been gradually enlarging. High kilovoltage x-rays of her neck demonstrate asymmetric narrowing of the subglottic region. What is the most likely diagnosis?**

A subglottic hemangioma.

O   **A 9 year old male presents with headaches and a rock hard left posterior triangle mass. Examination is significant for mouth breathing and bilateral serous otitis media. Fine needle aspiration of the neck mass reveals poorly differentiated malignant cells. What is the most likely source of the tumor?**

The nasopharynx.

O   **A 7 year old female presents for the evaluation of florid warty lesions growing from both tonsils. Biopsy demonstrates a well differentiated, nonkeratinizing squamous epithelium growing over a fibrovascular stalk. What is the most likely diagnosis?**

Papillomatosis.

O   **What etiology must be considered in the above patient?**

Sexual abuse.

O   *An 11 year old underwent excisional biopsy of a midline cyst adjacent to the hyoid bone. He continues to experience drainage and breakdown of his surgical wound. What is the treatment of choice?*

A Sistrunk procedure, the definitive procedure for thyroglossal duct cysts.

O   **A 6 month old female has experienced persistent mucinous drainage from a tiny pit at the angle of the mandible, for which surgical excision is recommended. What motor nerve is at risk?**

The facial nerve.

O   **An infant is born with a large port wine stain involving the forehead and maxilla. What other organ system should be evaluated?**

The central nervous system. Capillary malformations (port wine stains) involving the V1 and V2 distribution may be indicative of Sturge-Weber syndrome, with vascular malformations involving the brain, resulting in seizures and cognitive impairment.

O   **What percentage of thyroid nodules in children are malignant?**

25 to 55%.

O   **A 3 year old sustains bilateral subcondylar fractures of the mandible. Occlusion is normal and radiological studies demonstrate minimal displacement. What is the recommended management?**

A soft diet and physical therapy aimed at maintaining range of motion.

O   **An 11 year old boy struck his neck on a wire while riding an all-terrain vehicle. He is hoarse, has an abrasion directly over his thyroid cartilage and has neck and chest crepitus but is not in respiratory distress. After a complete history and physical examination, how is the airway assessed?**

Flexible laryngoscopy.

O   **What is the most common cause of acute facial paralysis in children?**

Bell's Palsy. However, in some series, it appears that Lyme Disease may be the most common.

O   **What is the immediate treatment of acute facial paralysis associated with otitis media?**

Myringotomy or myringotomy with tube insertion and appropriate antibiotics.

❍   **An 8 year old boy has a draining ear filled with friable tissue. CT demonstrates a punched out lytic lesion of the temporal bone. Biopsies show only lipid laden histiocytes. What is the most likely diagnosis?**

Histiocytosis X.

❍   **What is the immediate treatment for a tympanic membrane perforation caused by a cotton tipped applicator, in the absence of dizziness or hearing loss?**

Observation. Spontaneous healing occurs is approximately 90%.

❍   **What is the treatment for laryngomalacia in a 4 month old with adequate weight gain and no respiratory distress?**
Observation.

❍   *Posterior compression of the esophagus demonstrated on barium esophagogram is most likely caused by what vascular anomaly?*

An aberrant subclavian artery.

❍   **Tracheomalacia is most likely to cause stridor during which phase of respiration?**

Exhalation.

❍   **What physical features constitute the Pierre-Robin sequence?**

Glossoptosis, micrognathia and cleft palate.

❍   **A 4 month old male has a history of tracheo-esophageal fistula repaired successfully, as well as an imperforate anus. He has frequent choking and cyanosis with feeding. Barium swallow demonstrates free aspiration at the larynx. What is the best way to secure a diagnosis?**

Direct laryngoscopy. Laryngotracheo-esophageal clefts may be associated with tracheo-esophageal fistula and are likely to result in aspiration.

❍   **What is the pathophysiological difference of acid burns and alkaline burns in corrosive injuries of the esophagus?**

Acid causes a coagulative necrosis, which tends to protect the deeper tissues, as opposed to alkaline burns, which create a liquefactive necrosis and are associated with more extensive burns.

❍   **What medical therapy may be beneficial for patients with corrosive burns of the esophagus?**

Antibiotics hasten epithelialization and corticosteroids may decrease stricture formation.

❍   **A 4 month old child had a tracheotomy placed for vocal cord paralysis. He presents to the emergency room in severe respiratory distress. A suction catheter cannot be placed through the tracheotomy tube. What is the next step in management?**

Remove the tracheotomy tube. If possible, reinsert an identical or smaller replacement.

❍   **What are the leading causes of persistent cough in the newborn?**

Gastroesophageal reflux and airway anomalies.

❍   **T/F: Gastroesophageal reflux is thought to be one of the primary causes of sudden infant death syndrome.**

True.

❍   **What is the most likely etiology of bilateral vocal cord paralysis in the newborn?**

Central nervous system pathology, specifically hydrocephalus and the Arnold Chiari malformation.

❍   **An 8 French catheter is unable to be passed beyond 2.5 cm through either nare in a newborn with respiratory distress. What is the first step in airway management?**

Establishment of an oral airway.

❍   **T/F: Surgery of the nasal septum is contraindicated in young children.**

False.

❍   **A 3 year old with constant purulent nasal drainage and recurrent pneumonia has dextrocardia on chest x-ray. What is the most likely diagnosis?**

Kartagener's syndrome.

❍   **A 5 year old presents to the emergency room 5 days after having sustained a blow directly to the nasal tip. Although no nasal fracture is suspected, intranasal examination reveals a markedly widened, erythematous and boggy nasal septum. What is the appropriate treatment?**

Immediate drainage is necessary to prevent cartilage necrosis and loss of nasal support that would lead to a saddle nose deformity.

❍   **What are the components of the CHARGE sequence?**

Colobomata, heart defects, choanal atresia, retarded growth, genital hypoplasia and ear anomalies.

❍   **A 7 year old presents with fever, periorbital edema and erythema. She has had a cold for the last 6 days. Extraocular movements are subdued but intact. What is the appropriate management?**

Hospitalization and intravenous antibiotics. If symptoms progress over 24 hours, vision or extraocular motility begins to worsen, CT scanning should be performed and surgical drainage considered.

❍   **A 4 year old has constant nasal congestion. Examination reveals that both nasal cavities are obstructed by shiny, translucent tissue. What diagnostic test would be most helpful?**

Nasal polyps in a prepubescent child is highly suggestive of cystic fibrosis. A sweat chloride level should be obtained.

❍   **What is the most common source of bleeding in pediatric epistaxis?**

The anterior nasal septum in Kiesselbach's area.

GYNECOLOGY PEARLS

It is good to rub and polish our brain against that of others.
Michel de Montaigne

O   **What is the incidence of uterine sarcomas?**

2 to 4%.

O   **Prior pelvic irradiation is associated with the development of what type of uterine sarcoma?**

Malignant mixed mesodermal tumors (MMMT).

O   **What histologic criteria are used when diagnosing a benign endometrial stromal nodule?**

Proliferation of uniform, normal-appearing stromal cells with a well-circumscribed, noninfiltrative margin, absence of lymph-vascular space involvement and the mitotic count is usually less than 5 per 10 high power fields.

O   **How are endometrial stromal nodules treated?**

Hysterectomy is recommended. However, successful treatment using myomectomy has been reported.

O   **Worm-like extension of tumor into lymphatic and vascular channels, occasionally with extensive extrauterine extension is seen in what type of sarcoma?**

Low-grade endometrial stromal sarcomas. A similar pattern has been described for intravenous leiomyomatosis.

O   **Why is removal of the ovaries recommended for patients undergoing surgery for a low-grade stromal sarcoma?**

These tumors often have high levels of estrogen and progesterone receptors and their growth may be stimulated by estrogen.

O   **What percentage of stage I low-grade endometrial stromal sarcoma cases recur?**

50%.

O   **What is the most common neoplasm in reproductive-aged women?**

Benign leiomyomata.

O   **How does the origin of leiomyosarcomas differ from that of other uterine sarcomas?**

Leiomyosarcomas originate in the myometrium; all others originate in the endometrium.

O   **What is the average age for patients with leiomyosarcomas?**

53 years.

О   **A preoperative diagnosis of leiomyosarcoma is made in what percentage of cases?**
15%.

О   *What is the best predictor of recurrence-free interval for early stage leiomyosarcomas?*

The mitotic index.

О   **What is the effect of adjuvant radiation therapy on early stage leiomyosarcomas?**

Pelvic recurrences have been shown to be reduced by almost 50%.

О   **What histologic components must be present to make the diagnosis of a MMMT?**

Malignant epithelial and stromal components.

О   **What is the most common heterologous stromal component in a MMMT?**

Rhabdomyosarcoma.

О   **Surgical staging will upstage what percentage of patients with MMMT clinically confined to the uterus?**

25 to 50%.

О   **What is the incidence of recurrence in cases of uterine adenosarcoma?**

25%.

О   **What histologic features are associated with an increased risk of recurrence for stage I adenosarcoma?**

Sarcomatous overgrowth and deep myometrial invasion.

О   **What is the effect of estrogen on the endometrium?**

It causes the endometrial glands to lengthen and the glandular epithelium to become pseudostratified.

О   **In a woman of reproductive age, what is the first step in the evaluation of dysfunctional uterine bleeding following the history and physical examination?**

A pregnancy test.

О   **What is most common cause of dysfunctional uterine bleeding in adolescence?**

Anovulation.

О   **What percentage of adolescents that require hospitalization for abnormal bleeding have an underlying coagulation disorder?**

25%. The majority of these patients will have Von Willebrand's disease, problems with platelet number or problems with platelet function.

О   **What is the most common presenting complaint for a woman with cervical cancer?**

Menorrhagia.

О   **What is the normal thickness of the myometrium?**

1 to 2 cm.

○   **What is the most common cause of postmenopausal bleeding?**

Atrophic endometrium and/or atrophic vaginitis.

○   **What are most common causes of estrogen withdrawal bleeding?**

Bilateral oophorectomy, radiation of mature follicles and administration of estrogen to a previously oophorectomized woman followed by its withdrawal.

○   **Decline in what hormone heralds the onset of menses?**

Progesterone.

○   **Oral contraceptive use is associated with how much of a reduction in the risk of ovarian cancer?**

40% after 4 years and 60% after 12 years. There is a persistent protective effect after discontinuation of use.

○   **What is a second-degree prolapse of the uterus?**

The cervix has descended and is visible in but not protruding beyond, the introitus.

○   **What vascular event triggers shedding of the endometrium?**

Spasm of the spiral arteries resulting in ischemia of the tissue and sloughing.

○   **What is the embryologic origin of the fallopian tube?**

The paramesonephric duct.

○   **What is the site of most ectopic pregnancies?**

The fallopian ampulla.

○   **What functional ovarian cyst is most commonly associated with a hydatidiform mole?**

A theca lutein cyst.

○   **A 10 year old girl presents with an adnexal mass. What is the most common etiology?**

A mature cystic teratoma (dermoid cysts).

○   **A 6 year old girl presents for evaluation of premature thelarche. Her workup reveals Tanner stage 4 breast development, numerous cafe' au lait spots and ovarian cysts. What is the most likely diagnosis?**

McCune-Albright syndrome.

○   **What percentage of teratomas are bilateral?**

10 to 15%.

○   **What is the etiology of a mature teratoma?**

It arises from a single germ cell after the first meiotic division.

○   **What is the most common complication of teratomas?**

Torsion.

❍   **What is the risk of malignant transformation in a mature teratoma?**

Less than 2%.

❍   **What is the most common type of malignant transformation in a mature teratoma?**

Squamous cell carcinoma.

❍   **What percentage of patients with anovulation associated with polycystic ovarian disease do not have the expected reversal of the LH:FSH ratio?**

20 to 40%.

❍   **What is the most common benign, solid ovarian tumor?**

Fibroma.

❍   **A benign ovarian tumor is removed from a 50 year old female. The pathology report makes note of pale epithelial cells with a coffee bean nucleus. What is the most likely diagnosis?**

A brenner tumor.

❍   **A 43 year old female presents 5 years following a TAH/BSO for benign disease with a palpable pelvic mass and cyclical pelvic pain. The FSH level is in the premenopausal range. What is the most likely diagnosis?**

Ovarian remnant syndrome.

❍   **What is the risk of malignant degeneration in a leiomyoma?**

Less than 0.5%.

❍   **What is leiomyomatosis peritonealis disseminata?**

A rare condition in which benign leiomyomatous nodules are spread out over the pelvic and abdominal peritoneum. This usually occurs in young women and is associated with a recent pregnancy or estrinizing granulosa tumor.

❍   *When should PAP smears be initiated?*

When a woman becomes sexually active or reaches the age of 18 years.

❍   *How effective have PAP smears been in reducing the incidence of cervical cancer?*

It has decreased by almost 80%.

❍   **What is the false-negative rate for PAP smears?**

20%.

❍   **What is the most common presenting symptom for patients with cervical cancer?**

Abnormal vaginal bleeding.

❍   **What is the relative frequency of the two major histologic subtypes of cervical cancer?**

Squamous cell carcinoma occurs in 85 to 90% and adenocarcinoma accounts for the majority of the remaining cases.

❍   **Examination under anesthesia (EUA) reveals a 3 cm cervical carcinoma with left parametrial involvement not extending to the pelvic wall. The remainder of the staging evaluation is unremarkable. What stage is this patient's tumor?**

Stage IIb.

❍   **If the above patient also had hydronephrosis, what stage would her tumor be assigned?**

Stage IIIb.

❍   **What is the incidence of pelvic lymph node metastasis for stage Ib cervical cancer?**

15%.

❍   **For stage I cervical cancer, how does tumor size greater than 4 cm affect the incidence of pelvic lymph node metastasis?**

There is a three-fold increase.

❍   **What lymph node group is most frequently involved with metastatic cervical cancer?**

The external iliac group.

❍   **A coloposcopically directed cervical biopsy from a 25 year old femal G0 P0, reveals a small focus of invasive squamous cell carcinoma. What is the next step in this patient's management?**

Cervical cone biopsy.

❍   **The cardinal ligaments are exposed during a radical hysterectomy when what two pelvic spaces are developed?**

The paravesicle space anterior to the cardinal ligament and the pararectal space posteriorly.

❍   **Ureterovaginal fistulas occur in what percentage of patients undergoing radical hysterectomy?**

1 to 2%.

❍   **What is the incidence of small bowel obstruction following radiation used as primary therapy for cervical cancer?**

1 to 4%.

❍   **What are the advantages of radical hysterectomy over radiation therapy for stage I cervical cancer?**

Ovarian preservation, unimpaired vaginal function and establishment of extent of disease.

❍   **How does a modified radical hysterectomy differ from a radical hysterectomy?**

The uterine artery is divided medial to the ureter rather than at its origin, the cardinal ligament is divided medial to the ureter rather than at the pelvic wall, only the medial portion of the uterosacral ligament is resected and the vaginal margin is smaller.

○   **Clinical staging of a 56 year old female with cervical cancer involving the left parametrium detects a 6 cm complex right adnexal mass. How is treatment affected by the mass?**

Surgical exploration is necessary to exclude a simultaneous ovarian cancer with staging or debulking as indicated. Given the parametrial extension, a hysterectomy should not be performed.

○   **When invasive cervical cancer is incidentally discovered following a simple hysterectomy, what is the most common preoperative diagnosis?**

Cervical dysplasia.

○   **What is the 1-year survival rate following cervical cancer recurrence?**

15%.

○   **What is the therapy of choice for an isolated vaginal cuff recurrence following radical hysterectomy for cervical cancer?**

External beam radiation therapy followed by brachytherapy.

○   **What clinical triad is strongly indicative of disease extension to the pelvic wall?**

Unilateral leg edema, sciatic pain and ureteral obstruction.

○   **What is the best predictor that endometrial hyperplasia will progress to endometrial carcinoma?**

The presence or absence of cytologic atypia.

○   **What is the most common clinical condition associated with the development of endometrial hyperplasia?**

Polycystic ovary syndrome.

○   **Hyperplasia with cytologic atypia, treated with progesterone, will progress to cancer in what percentage of cases?**

25 to 30%.

○   **In the postmenopausal woman, what is the main circulating estrogen?**

Estrone.

○   **What are the most common presenting symptoms of endometrial hyperplasia in a woman of reproductive age?**

Menorrhagia, metorrhagia and prolonged menses.

○   **What percentage of women will have endometrial hyperplasia on biopsy performed for abnormal or postmenopausal bleeding?**

8 to 9%.

○   **What differentiates complex atypical hyperplasia from well-differentiated adenocarcinoma?**

The presence of stromal invasion.

○   **What surgical options are currently available for the treatment of endometrial hyperplasia?**

Curettage for acute bleeding, hysteroscopy to exclude polyps and carcinoma and hysterectomy, particularly if cytologic atypia is present.

○   **What is the survival rate for women with a diagnosis of endometrial carcinoma confined to the uterus at the time of surgical staging?**

75%.

○   **What risk factors are associated with endometrial carcinoma?**

Obesity, nulliparity, early menarche and late menopause. Women 21 to 50 pounds over ideal body weight increase their risk of developing endometrial carcinomas three-fold. Women in excess of 50 pounds over ideal body weight increase their chance of developing endometrial carcinoma ten-fold.

○   **What is type II Lynch syndrome?**

A hereditary predisposition to the development of colon, breast, ovarian and endometrial cancer.

○   **Who might benefit from endometrial cancer screening?**

Postmenopausal women on exogenous unopposed estrogen, obese postmenopausal women, women whose menopause occurred after age 52 and premenopausal women with chronic anovulation.

○   **What effect does the prior use of oral contraceptive agents have on the development of endometrial cancer?**

It decreases the risk.

○   **What is the most common presenting complaint of a woman with endometrial cancer?**

Dysfunctional uterine bleeding.

○   **What is the initial workup for a woman whose history is suspicious for endometrial cancer?**

Pelvic examination, PAP smear, biopsy of any abnormal cervical or vaginal lesions and endometrial biopsy.

○   **In what clinical circumstances are pelvic and abdominal CT helpful in evaluating patients with endometrial cancer on biopsy?**

Abnormal liver function tests, hepatomegaly, palpable upper abdominal mass, palpable extrauterine pelvic disease and ascites.

○   **How does endometrial carcinoma spread?**

Direct extension to adjacent structures, transtubal passage of exfoliated cells, lymphatic dissemination and hematogenous dissemination.

○   **Why do younger women have a better prognosis for endometrial carcinoma compared to older women?**

Young women tend to have lower grade tumors with less myometrial invasion.

○   **What is the significance of estrogen and progesterone receptor status in the prognosis of women with a diagnosis of endometrial carcinoma?**

ER status does not correlate well with prognosis but the absence of progesterone receptors is associated with a poor prognosis.

O   **What is the estrogen and progesterone receptor status in obese women with endometrial cancer?**

The majority are ER+ and PR+.

O   **What is a Walthard nest?**

A benign inclusion cyst created in the fallopian tube by invagination of the tubal serosa.

O   **What is the most common benign tumor of the fallopian tubes?**
Adenomatoid tumors (benign mesotheliomas).

O   **What histologic finding is associated with carcinoma in situ (CIS) of the fallopian tube?**

Cytologically malignant and mitotically active nuclei, with or without the formation of papillae by the endosalpingeal epithelial cells.

O   **What tumor marker is useful in the follow-up of tubal serous carcinomas?**

CA-125.

O   **What is the most common primary malignant neoplasm of the fallopian tubes?**

Papillary serous adenocarcinoma.

O   **What is the standard treatment for tubal carcinoma?**

Total abdominal hysterectomy and bilateral salpingo-oophorectomy (TAH/BSO), aggressive cytoreductive surgery and chemotherapy.

O   **How does depth of invasion relate to survival in fallopian tube carcinomas?**

Depth of invasion is inversely related to survival.

O   **What is the lymphatic drainage of the fallopian tubes?**

The paraaortic lymph nodes.

O   **What is the most common type of tubal sarcoma?**

Leiomyosarcoma.

O   **What risk factors have been linked with vulvar cancer?**

Advancing postmenopausal age, hypertension, diabetes, obesity and smoking.

O   **What link does the human papilloma virus (HPV) have with vulvar cancer?**

HPV DNA can be identified in about 70 to 80% of intraepithelial lesions but is seen in only 10 to 50% of invasive lesions. HPV type 16 seems to be most common but types 6 and 33 have also been identified.

O   **What is the name and location of the last node of the deep femoral nodal group?**

The cloquet node (sentinel node). It is located just beneath Poupart's ligament.

O   **What vulvar lesion has the classic cake-icing effect secondary to hyperemic areas associated with a superficial white coating?**

Paget's disease of the vulva.

❍ **What is the treatment of Paget's disease without an underlying adenocarcinoma?**

This is a true intraepithelial neoplasia and can be treated as such with wide local excision.

❍ **What are the most frequent histologic subtypes seen in Bartholin gland cancer?**

Adenocarcinoma and squamous cell carcinoma.

❍ **What is the most frequent primary vulvar sarcoma?**
Leiomyosarcoma.

❍ **What is the most common location on the vulva to find an adenoid cystic carcinoma?**

Bartholin's gland.

❍ **What is the single most important prognostic factor in women with vulvar cancer?**

Lymph node metastases.

❍ **What are the most common complications associated with radical vulvectomy?**

Wound breakdown and lymphedema.

❍ **Prior to treatment of Paget's disease of the vulva, what screening tests should be performed?**

Breast exam, mammography and cytologic and colposcopic evaluation of the cervix, vagina and vulva.

❍ **What vaginal tumor presents as a mass of grape-like nodules most commonly in the first 2 years of life?**

Embryonal rhabdomyosarcoma (sarcoma botryoides).

❍ **What is the most common vaginal tumor?**

Secondary carcinoma from extension of a cervical cancer.

❍ **What is the most common type of primary vaginal cancer?**

Squamous cell.

❍ **What is the most common location of a primary vaginal carcinoma lesion?**

The upper third and posterior wall of the vagina.

❍ **What is the most frequent presenting symptom of vaginal cancer?**

Vaginal discharge.

❍ **What is the primary mode of therapy for vaginal cancer?**

Radiation therapy.

❍ **What is the treatment of clear cell adenocarcinoma confined to the upper vagina and/or cervix?**

Radical hysterectomy with upper vaginectomy and pelvic lymphadenectomy with retention of the ovaries.

O   **What is the treatment of malignant melanoma of the vagina?**

Radical excision with nodal dissection.

O   **What is the peak age at presentation of a DES-related clear cell adenocarcinoma of the vagina or cervix?**

About 19 years.

O   **What association has been described between the risk of developing vaginal cancer and the time of first exposure to DES?**

The risk was greatest for those exposed the first 16 weeks in utero and declined for those whose exposure began in the 17th week or later.

O   **What is the incidence of clear cell adenocarcinoma in women prenatally exposed to DES?**

1.4 per 1000.

O   **How is fetal compromise during nonobstetric surgery managed?**

Exaggerated left uterine displacement, administration of a higher inspired concentration of oxygen, adjustment of maternal ventilation, augmentation of maternal circulating blood volume and pharmacologic treatment of hypotension.

O   **What percentage of patients with pelvic inflammatory disease (PID) become infertile?**

10%.

O   **What are the risk factors for PID?**

Age less than 20, multiple sexual partners, nulliparity and previous history of PID.

O   **What is the most likely diagnosis in a patient whose uterus is larger than expected from the history of gestation, has vaginal bleeding and passes grape-like tissue from the vagina?**

Hydatidiform mole.

O   **What are chocolate cysts?**

Endometriomas (cystic forms of endometriosis on the ovary).

O   **What is Meig's syndrome?**

Ascites with hydrothorax associated with benign ovarian tumors with fibrous elements, usually fibromas.

O   **What is the treatment for recurrent cervical cancer?**

External- and internal-beam radiotherapy or pelvic exenteration.

O   **What are the risk factors for vulvar carcinoma?**

Older age, smoking, previous squamous cell carcinoma of the cervix or vagina, chronic vulvar dystrophy and immunocompromise.

O   **What is the method of spread of vulvar carcinoma?**

Lymphatic (to the inguinal nodes).

○   **What is the treatment of choice for vulvar carcinoma?**

Radical vulvectomy with inguinal lymphadenectomy.

○   **What are the indications for dilation and curettage?**

Removal of an endometrial polyp or hydatid mole, termination of pregnancy/incomplete abortion, removal of retained placental tissue and relief of profuse uterine hemorrhage.

○   **What major complication is associated with dilation and curettage?**

Perforation of the uterus.

○   **What muscles constitute the urogenital diaphragm?**

The ischiocavernosus, bulbocavernosus and transverse perinei.

○   **What is the blood supply to the pelvis?**

The internal iliac arteries and the middle sacral artery.

○   **What are the most common organisms that cause pelvic inflammatory disease?**

N. gonorrhea and chlamydia.

○   **What is thought to be the cause of endometriosis?**

Retrograde menstruation.

○   **What are the risk factors for carcinoma of the cervix?**

Multiple sexual partners, early age at first intercourse and early first pregnancy.

○   **By what route do cervical cancers usually spread?**

Predominantly by lymphatic channels.

○   **What is the treatment for patients with Stage IB and IIA cervical cancer?**

Radical hysterectomy with pelvic lymphadenectomy or definitive radiotherapy.

○   **In the treatment of cervical cancer, when is it required to use combination radiotherapy and surgery?**

With Stage IB and cancers that exceed 5 cm in diameter.

○   **When is extended-field radiotherapy required?**

When metastases are found in the common iliac or paraaortic lymph nodes.

HEMATOLOGY AND ONCOLOGY PEARLS

Fever, the eternal reproach to the physician.
John Milton

○ **When do cells die after treatment with radiation?**

Usually at the time of cell division.

○ **Carcinoembryonic antigen (CEA) is found in what fetal tissues?**

The gastrointestinal tract, liver and pancreas.

○ **T/F: Prostatic acid phosphatase is secreted by the normal prostate.**

True.

○ **CA 15.3 is elevated in patients with what tumors?**

Breast, ovary and lung.

○ **What factors affect the risk of long-term injury from radiation?**

The type and amount of tissue treated, the total dose of radiation and the dose given with each daily fraction.

○ **What are the primary reasons for fractionation of radiation doses?**

To allow for repair, redistribtion, reoxygenation and repopulation of cells.

○ **To which platelet glycoprotein does Von Willebrand factor bind to enhance platelet aggregation?**

Glycoprotein Ib.

○ *Fibrinogen forms bridges between activated platelets by binding to which platelet glycoprotein?*

Glycoprotein IIb/IIIa.

○ **What is the characteristic chromosomal abnormality seen in patient with Burkitt's lymphoma?**

A chromosomal translocation (8:14).

○ **Beta-napthlyamine is associated with what neoplasm?**

Bladder cancer.

○ **Activated factor X, (Xa), in combination with which two cofactors, activates prothrombin on the surface of platelets?**

Ionized calcium and factor Va.

O   **What complex activates protein C on the surface of endothelial cells?**

Thrombin-thrombomodulin complex.

O   **What is the most central natural anticoagulant protein?**

Antithrombin III.

O   **What are the major endogenous activators of plasminogen?**

Tissue plasminogen activator (tPA) and urokinase.

O   **What fragments are released when fibrin is digested by plasmin?**

One molecule of fragment E and two (separate) molecules of fragment D.

O   **What intrinsic factors (other than above) activate plasminogen?**

Factor XII, prekallikrein and high-molecular-weight kininogen.

O   **Circulating neutrophils and monocytes interact with platelets through which molecule?**

P-selectin.

O   *When should heparin-induced thrombocytopenia be suspected?*

When thrombosis occurs while receiving heparin or when there is a fall in the platelet count to less than 100,000/ul.

O   **What are the molecular events in heparin-induced thrombocytopenia?**

It is believed to be caused by a heparin-dependent IgG platelet antibody that causes aggregation of platelets when exposed to heparin.

O   *What is the nature of the thromboses in heparin-induced thrombocytopenia?*

It can be arterial or venous and is a characteristic white clot.

O   **T/F: Changing from bovine derived heparin to porcine derived heparin is sufficient therapy for a patient with heparin-induced thrombocytopenia.**

False.

O   **What is the typical presentation of a patient with antithrombin III deficiency?**

Homozygotes usually die in infancy and 85% of heterozygotes have suffered a thrombotic event by 50 years of age. The diagnosis should be suspected in a patient with a thrombotic event while on heparin or an inability to be anticoagulated with heparin.

O   **T/F: This disorder can be acquired.**

True.

O   **What are the common causes of acquired antithrombin III deficiency?**

Liver disease, malignancy, nephrotic syndrome, DIC, malnutrition or increased protein catabolism.

O   *What is the appropriate therapy for a patient with antithrombin III deficiency, requiring anticoagulation?*

Fresh frozen plasma (FFP) can be used as a source of antithrombin III when heparin is necessary, followed by anticoagulation with sodium warfarin. Additionally, antithrombin III concentrates are available.

O   **What is Krukenberg's tumor?**

An ovarian mass detectable on bimanual pelvic examination that represents a drop metastasis or transcoelomic implantation of the ovary from an intraabdominal site (classically the stomach).

O   *How does sodium warfarin (Coumadin) work as an anticoagulant?*

It prevents the reduction of vitamin K once it has functioned as a cofactor for the carboxylation of factors II, VII, IX and X.

O   *What is the danger of initiating anticoagulation with coumadin alone?*

Coumadin may decrease protein C levels prior to a reduction in clotting factors, thereby inducing a pro-coagulant state in the early phases of therapy.

O   *When is this situation particularly devastating?*

In patients with protein C deficiency, coumadin can cause an excessive reduction in protein C levels. The resulting pro-coagulant state can cause skin necrosis, usually in fatty regions such as the breasts, buttocks or thighs, from clotting in the microcirculation.

O   **T/F: Cancer cells proliferate faster than normal cells.**

False.

O   *What is the molecular abnormality in resistance to activated protein C?*

It is most likely due to a decrease in the anticoagulant function of factor V (autosomal dominant, factor V leiden mutation).

O   **What is the most common laboratory abnormality associated with the antiphospholipid syndrome?**

An elevated aPTT not corrected by normal plasma, in the face of other standard coagulation tests that are normal.

O   **T/F: A patient with thrombosis associated with the antiphospholipid syndrome may receive heparin therapy.**

True. Proper treatment includes heparinization followed by long-term sodium warfarin therapy

O   *What laboratory abnormalities are associated with hemophilia A?*

Prolongation of aPTT with other tests being normal.

O   **What is the minimum level of factor VIII required for hemostasis?**

30%.

O   **What is the molecular abnormality in hemophilia B?**

An X-linked recessive deficiency of factor IX (Christmas Factor).

O   **T/F: Hemophilia A is clinically distinguishable from hemophilia B.**

False.

O   **Which clotting factors, labile factors, are most likely to be decreased as a result of massive transfusion?**

Factors V and VIII (low half lives).

O   **T/F: Cyclophosphamide is an appropriate drug for intraperitoneal administration.**

False.

O   *What is the mechanism of action of methotrexate?*

It binds dihydrofolate reductase, preventing reduction of folate to tetrahydrofolate, which is necessary for production of thymidine and purines.

O   **What is the maximum total cumulative dose of adriamycin suggested to minimize the risk of cardiomyopathy?**

450 to 550 mg/m2.

O   **What immediate steps should be taken to minimize tissue damage following extravasation of adriamycin?**

Stop the infusion, aspirate the drug from the site, if possible, and apply ice to the affected area.

O   **What types of chromosomal abnormalities are found in tumors?**

Reciprocal translocation, deletional abnormalities and increased DNA.

O   **What is the treatment for primary mediastinal seminomas?**

Radio- or chemotherapy.

O   *What tumor marker is associated with choriocarcinomas?*

Beta-HCG.

O   *What is the mechanism of action of paclitaxel?*

Enhancement of tubulin polymerization.

O   **Serum albumin levels may be predictive of what toxicity associated with ifosfamide?**

Central nervous system toxicity may occur with serum albumin levels less than 3.5 mg/dl.

O   *What antibiotics should be used initially in a febrile neutropenic patient?*

Drug combinations including gram-negative coverage (aminoglycosides or aztreonam) and an extended spectrum penicillin or cephalosporin.

O   **What is the treatment for chemotherapy induced mucositis?**

Topical solutions containing viscous xylocaine, antacids and antifungals may be used along with adequate pain relief.

❍ **What is vincristine belly?**

Constipation caused by autonomic neuropathy secondary to vincristine.

❍ **What drug is usually associated with the hemolytic-uremic syndrome?**

Mitomycin C.

❍ **What is the dose-limiting toxicity of paclitaxel?**

Myelosuppression.

❍ **What is the term for the use of cisplatin concurrently with radiation for primary therapy of cervical cancer?**

Radiosensitization.

❍ *What factors shift the oxygen curve to the right?*

CADET step right. High CO2, Acidosis, high DPG, Increase temp.

❍ **What is the only clotting factor not made in liver?**

Factor 8.

❍ **How long will ASA affect the platelet?**

7 days the entire life of the platelet, because it irreversibly binds cyclooxygenase.

❍ **What clotting abnormalities are found with VW disease?**

Long PTT and long bleeding time or functional platelet assay.

❍ **VW disease is treated with what?**

Recombinant factor VIII or cryoprecipitate. However type I and type III have low vwf and often respond to DDAVP. Type II - the platelets are poor quality.

❍ **What is the treatment for Hodgkin's disease?**

Combination chemotherapy, such as nitrogen **m**ustard, vincristine (**O**ncovin), **p**rocarbazine and **p**redinsone (MOPP) or MOPP/ABV (**a**driamycin, **b**leomycin and **v**inblastine).

❍ **What are the most commonly used drug(s) for primary treatment of advanced ovarian cancer?**

Paclitaxel and either cisplatin or carboplatin.

❍ **What is the dose limiting toxicity of Topotecan?**

Myelosuppression.

❍ **Can LMWH cause HIT?**

Yes.

O   **What is involved in Phase III of clinical testing of new drugs?**

Agents that have demonstrated a benefit (in Phase II) are compared in a randomized fashion with standard treatment programs.

O   **What is the most commonly used drug as a single agent for gestational trophoblastic neoplasia?**

Methotrexate.

O   **What drugs are used for prevention of hypersensitivity reactions associated with paclitaxel?**

Corticosteroids and H1 and H2 blockers.

O   *What is the dose limiting toxicity associated with Vincristine?*

Neurotoxicity.

O   **Why is mesna used in conjunction with ifosfamide?**

To prevent hemorrhagic cystitis.

O   **T/F: Patients with ovarian cancer can be followed by serial evaluation of CA 125 levels.**

False; it is not specific enough.

O   **What is the mechanism of action of vinca alkaloid type drugs?**

Binding of tubulin to produce mitotic arrest.

O   **T/F: Cyclophosphamide is specific for the M phase of the cell cycle.**

False.

O   **T/F: Methotrexate is primarily excreted by the kidneys.**

True.

O   **What is the dose limiting toxicity of 5-FU?**

Stomatitis, often with nausea and vomiting.

O   **Actinomycin D is frequently used as a single agent for therapy of what gynecologic malignancy?**

Gestational trophoblastic neoplasms.

O   *What is the most significant side effect associated with bleomycin?*

Interstitial pnuemonitis.

O   **Interstitial pneumonitis resulting from bleomycin can be measured by what parameter of pulmonary function testing?**

Decreased diffusion capacity.

O   **What is the dose limiting toxicity associated with hydroxyurea?**

Myelosuppression.

❍ **What is the mechanism of action of actinomycin D?**

It blocks RNA synthesis by intercalating DNA nucleotide pairs.

❍ **T/F: Patients who are HIV positive are at increased risk for developing Hodgkin's disease.**

False, but true for NHL.

❍ **What is irradiation recall?**

Skin erythema and irritation in a previously irradiated field following administration of chemotherapy. Adriamycin and actinomycin D are commonly reported.

❍ **Cerebellar ataxia is associated with what chemotherapeutic agent?**

5-FU.

❍ **What type of blotting technique is used to analyze protein structure?**

A Western blot.

❍ **What is the dose limiting toxicity of carboplatin?**

Myelosuppression.

❍ **Why does tumor heterogeneity often result in drug resistance?**

Spontaneous mutations give rise to small numbers of resistant cells that may rapidly reproduce when sensitive cells are killed.

❍ **What is the MDR gene?**

The Multiple Drug Resistance gene is normally present in some human tissues and may be activated in tumors by exposure to certain chemotherapeutic agents, resulting in resistance to many drugs.

❍ **Adriamycin-associated cardiotoxicity may be anticipated by the use of what imaging study?**

A MUGA scan.

❍ **What is the most important factor in predicting the efficacy of progestin therapy in endometrial cancer?**

Progesterone receptor status of the tumor.

❍ **What systemic chemotherapeutic agents are used for Stage IV colon cancer?**

5-FU and leucovorin.

❍ **5-FU has been used in a topical form for the treatment of what condition?**

Multifocal vaginal intraepithelial neoplasia.

❍ **Patients undergoing surgery after bleomycin treatment should avoid high inhaled oxygen concentrations. Why?**

Acute pulmonary decompensation can occur.

O   **What finding on a peripheral blood smeer is characteristic of surgical or functional splenectomy?**

Howell-Jolly bodies.

O   **T/F: The red blood cell distribution width (RDW) is elavated in patients with mechanical cardiac valves.**

True, secondary to production of fragmented cells.

O   **What type of anemia may be seen with Epstein-Barr virus?**

Aplastic anemia.

O   **What is the storage form of iron?**

Ferritin.

O   **What are the common complications of hereditary spherocytosis?**

Sphenic rupture, cholelithiasis and aplastic anemia.

O   **What type of hemolytic anemia is associated with ulcerative colitis?**

Autoimmune hemolytic anemia.

O   **What is the expected increase in the plalelet count following transfusion with 6 plalelet packs?**

40,000 to 50,000/mm^3.

IMMUNOLOGY AND TRANSPLANTATION PEARLS

The wise man mourns less for what age takes away then what it leaves behind.
William Wordsworth

❍ **What is an orthotopic graft?**

A graft placed in the anatomic position normally occupied by such tissue.

❍ **What chromosome contains the major histocompatibility complex (MHC)?**

Chromosome 6.

❍ **Which MHC antigens best trigger the proliferation of allogenic lymphocytes?**

Human leukocyte antigen (HLA) class II antigens (HLA-D, DR, DQ and DW/DR).

❍ *What cells have HLA Class I molecules?*

All nucleated cells.

❍ *What cells have HLA Class II molecules?*

Macrophages, dendritic cells, B cells and activated T cells.

❍ **T/F: Interferons (IFN-alpha, IFN-beta and IFN-gamma) induce increased expression of Class I molecules.**

True.

❍ **What cells produce IFN-alpha?**

Fibroblasts.

❍ **What is the action of oxytocin?**

It stimulates uterine contraction during labor and elicits milk ejection by myoepithelial cells of the mammary ducts.

❍ **What are the methods of determining the degree of histocompatibility between donor and recipient?**

MHC matching and mixed lymphocyte culture (MLC).

❍ **What is the most common use of the MLC?**

Related bone-marrow transplantation.

O   **What triggers the rejection reaction after transplantation?**

The immune response to the HLA antigens on the cells of the transplanted organ/tissue.

O   **What are the critical cytokines that influence lineage maturation?**

Granulocyte-macrophage colony stimulating factor (GM-CSF), interleukin-1 (IL-1) and erythropoietin.

O   **What is the clinical use of GM-CSF?**

It decreases infection in neutropenic patients.

O   **What organs are considered secondary lymphoid organs?**

The spleen, peripheral lymph nodes, skin and Peyer's patches.

O   **What constitutes the T-cell receptor complex (CD3)?**

The T cell's membrane-bound T-cell receptor (TCR) and associated transmembrane proteins.

O   *What T cell cluster of differentiation (CD) antigen lyses target cells and kills cells infected with virus?*

CD8.

O   **T/F: Mature T cells can reenter the thymus.**

False.

O   **What is required for a lymphocyte to become sensitized?**

An accessory antigen-presenting cell (APC) of the monocyte-macrophage line.

O   **What is the function of IL-2 with regard to the immune cellular response?**

It amplifies the immune response by exerting an autocrine feedback on the same cell and a paracrine effect to activate other T cells in the local microenvironment.

O   **What do antigen-stimulated B cells require to proliferate and produce antibody?**

T-helper cytokines.

O   **What T-cell subgroup inhibits the development of antibody-producing B cells and the generation of T-helper cells?**

T-suppressor cells.

O   **ABO incompatibility is an example of what type of hypersensitivity reaction?**

Type II.

O   **What cells do Class II alloantigens preferentially stimulate?**

CD4 and T-helper cells.

O   **What is the function of perforin (released by sensitized T cells)?**

It forms tubular transmembrane pores (once the cytotoxic T cell binds to the antigen on the target cell) to allow unidirectional granule exocytosis with destruction of the target cell.

❍ **T/F: IL-1 is cytotoxic for tumor cells.**

True.

❍ *What are the effects of tumor necrosis factor (TNF)?*

It acts synergistically with IL-1 to mediate acute-phase changes, including tumor necrosis, hypotension and inflammatory reactions.

❍ **What are the macrophage-derived cytokines?**

IL-1, Il-6 and TNF-alpha.

❍ **T/F: Circulating antibody is an obligatory participant in the rejection of solid tissue allografts.**

False.

❍ **How do antibodies activate the complement pathway?**

When an antibody binds to antigen, the antibody undergoes a conformational change that activates the constant (Fc) end of the antibody, which then triggers complement activation.

❍ **T/F: Complement mediates lytic destruction of antibody-bound cells.**

True.

❍ **What are the biologic actions of C3a?**

It causes release of histamine from mast cells, is chemotactic for PMNs, has a kinin activity and causes immune adherence.

❍ **What initiates release of cellular tissue thromboplastin?**

Damage to the endothelial cell membrane by antibody and complement or through the direct cytotoxic effects of lymphocytes.

❍ **What factor initiates the intrinsic pathway of the clotting system?**

Hageman factor (factor XII).

❍ **What is thought to be the etiology of the progressive, obliterative vascular reaction seen in a chronically rejecting allograft?**

A by-product of fibrin laid down along the endothelium that has been damaged by immune mechanisms.

❍ **How is the kinin system activated?**

By activation of Hageman factor, leading to the formation of kallikrein.

❍ **What characteristics of rejection are modified by immunosuppression agents?**

Endothelial cell damage in the allograft, hypertrophy and hyperplasia.

❍ **What are the characteristics of accelerated atherosclerosis?**

A thickened intimal layer with loss of the smooth endothelial lining, presence of vacuolated cells and a narrowed lumen.

○   **What is the role of platelets is allograft rejection?**

Platelet aggregation leads to release of histamine and serotonin, which increases capillary permeability. This results in exposure of the basement membrane and enhancement of platelet aggregation. Platelets also release factors that increase destruction.

○   **What is the only tissue that can be transplanted without chronic immunosuppression?**

Bone marrow stem cells.

○   *What is the mechanism of action of azathioprine (AZ)?*

It is a purine analog (antimetabolite) that interferes with DNA synthesis.

○   *What is the mechanism of action of FK 506?*

It inhibits T-cell activation and maturation.

○   **How does irradiation suppress the immune response?**

By preventing the differentiation and division of immunocompetent lymphocytes.

○   **How do alkylating agents suppress the immune response?**

They combine with DNA and other cellular components to prevent proliferation of immunocompetent cells.

○   **When are antimetabolites given to a transplant patient?**

At the time of transplantation and then for the life of the graft.

○   **What is the mechanism of action of AZ?**

It is structurally similar to inosine monophosphate, thus, it inhibits the enzymes that convert inosine nucleotide to adenosine and guanosine monophosphate. AZ also slows down the entire purine biosynthetic pathway by fraudulent feedback inhibition of cellular synthesis of RNA, DNA, cofactors and other active nucleotides.

○   **What is the role of methotrexate in chronic immunosuppression?**

It is used clinically only for bone marrow transplantation if there is a contraindication to cyclosporine or FK 506 as graft-versus-host (GVH) prophylaxis because of its severe toxicity.

○   **What is the mechanism of action of alkylating agents?**

They contain unstable rings with electron-seeking points that combine with electron-rich nucleophile groups (i.e., $-NH_2$, $-COOH$, $-SH$ and $-PO_3H_2$) and result in alkylation of DNA and RNA.

○   **What are the clinical uses of cyclophosphamide?**

It is used in renal transplant patients when liver toxicity prohibits the use of AZ and for bone marrow recipients.

○   **What side effects are specific to cyclophosphamide?**

Prompt fluid retention, severe hemorrhagic cystitis and cardiac toxicity.

❍   **What combination of drugs provides the most effective immunosuppression with the fewest side effects?**

Cyclosporine, prednisone and/or AZ.

❍   **What are the adverse effects of cyclosporine?**

Hirsutism, neurotoxicity, hyperkalemia, nephrotoxicity, hypertension and tremors.

❍   **T/F: Cyclosporine is effective against activated T cells.**

False.

❍   **T/F: The potency of FK 506 is much greater than that of cyclosporine.**

False.

❍   **How does FK 506 affect the immune response?**

It inhibits production of IL-2 and IFN-gamma.

❍   *What is the effect of adrenal corticosteroids on lymphocytes?*

Inhibition of DNA, RNA and protein synthesis as well as inhibition of glucose and amino acid transport.

❍   *What are the characteristics of chronic steroid administration?*

A cushingoid appearance, hypertension, weight gain, peptic ulcers, gastrointestinal bleeding, euphoric personality changes, cataract formation, hyperglycemia, diabetes, osteoporosis and avascular necrosis of bone.

❍   *What is the prototypic monoclonal antibody in clinical immunosuppression?*

OKT3.

❍   **What is the most important mode of cellular damage from radiation?**

Production of scattered breaks in the deoxyribose-phosphate backbone of DNA.

❍   *In what stage(s) of the cell cycle is radiation most effective?*

The M and G2 phase. (Lymphocytes are also sensitive in the G0 phase.)

❍   **What is the most common cause of death in transplant recipients?**

Infection.

❍   **The majority of deaths in transplant recipients are due to what organisms?**

Candida albicans, followed by aspergillus.

❍   *What are the most common viral organisms causing rejection in renal transplant patients?*

The herpes group DNA viruses (particularly CMV).

❍   **What percentage of renal transplant patients are infected with cytomegalovirus (CMV)?**

50 to 90%.

O   **What are the typical manifestations of CMV infection in transplant patients?**

A mild febrile illness followed by an antibody response and regression of viral symptoms.

O   **What are the most effective precautions for decreasing the number of severe infections?**

1.   Elimination of all sources of infection prior to transplantation.
2.   Proper technical procedures and gentle handling of tissues.
3.   Well-matched organs.
4.   Prevention of leukopenia (e.g., careful monitoring of AZ).

O   **What are the most frequent malignancies seen in transplant patients?**

Those that are common to immunosuppressed patients. Most are epithelial or lymphoid in origin (i.e., carcinoma in situ of the cervix, carcinoma of the lip, squamous or basal cell carcinoma of the skin and B cell lymphoma).

O   **What is the incidence of lymphoma in transplant recipients?**

350 times the average population.

O   **What percentage of transplant patients with lymphoma have brain involvement?**

50%.

O   **What is thought to be the etiology of lymphoma in transplant patients?**

Infection with Ebstein-Barr virus (EBV) (lymphoproliferative disease) (LPD).

O   **What is the etiology of hypertension in transplant patients?**

Prednisone, failure to regulate normal salt and water balance and secretion of renin.

O   **What is the critical period of ischemia after which extremity replantation is unsuccessful?**

There is no definite time, however, it appears that successful replantation of a limb can occur after 12 hours of ischemia and up to 36 hours for a finger.

O   **T/F: Motor nerve recovery is more successful in the ulnar nerve than in the median nerve.**

False.

O   **Removal of T cells from bone marrow grafts would theoretically eliminate the GVH reaction. Why is this not tolerated?**

T cells must be present to help the pluripotent bone marrow stem cells to engraft.

O   *What are the clinical manifestations of the GVH reaction?*

Skin rash, hepatic dysfunction, diarrhea, wasting and myelosuppression.

O   **How is the diagnosis of GVH reaction confirmed?**

Skin biopsy.

○ **What is the treatment for GVH reaction?**

FK 506 or cyclosporin plus steroids.

○ **T/F: Transplantation of insulin-producing islet cells (beta cells) is sufficient to achieve glucose hemostasis.**

True.

○ **T/F: Islet cell grafts are less antigenic than whole organ grafts.**

False.

○ **T/F: Islet cell graft rejection is accelerated compared to whole organ grafts.**

True. (Especially is diabetics, secondary to autoimmunity.)

○ **Why is there such interest in islet cell grafts when they have such dismal success rates?**

When the rejection reaction is overcome, there is no better way to improve the vascular and neurologic lesions of diabetes.

○ **What are the surgical approaches to pancreatic duct drainage?**

Bladder drainage, ductal injection with a synthetic polymer and enteric drainage.

○ **Why is bladder drainage the most favored?**

Because amylase levels rise early in pancreatic graft rejection and can be easily detected in the urine, in addition to it being the most successful technique.

○ **What is the survival of pancreatic grafts at 36 months?**

Greater than 60%.

○ **What is the most common type of patient population receiving small bowel transplants?**

Pediatric patients who have lost their small bowel secondary to malrotation with midgut volvulus or necrotizing enterocolitis (NEC).

○ **What patients require a liver transplant along with small bowel transplantation?**

Those who have been on long-term hyperalimentation with subsequent development of cirrhosis and liver failure.

○ **What are the most common liver diseases for which liver transplantation is required?**

Chronic active hepatitis (27%), followed by cholestatic liver disease (21%), biliary atresia (16.7%) and alcoholic cirrhosis (8.5%).

○ **T/F: Alcoholism is a contraindication to liver transplantation.**

True; unless the patient has abstained from alcohol for at least 2 years.

○ **T/F: Patients with active ulcerative colitis are excluded from liver transplantation.**

True.

❍   **What is the infectious work-up for a potential liver recipient?**

Chest x-ray, cultures of the blood, urine, throat, feces and ascites, hepatitis screen and a dental consult.

❍   **How is patency of the portal system evaluated prior to liver transplantation?**

CT, ultrasound and/or celiac angiography.

❍   **What are the most important systems to optimize prior to liver transplantation?**

Nutrition and pulmonary.

❍   **What precautions should be taken to minimize technical difficulties in liver transplantation?**

1.   Do not remove the spleen.
2.   Minimize dissection in the retroperitoneum and near the distal common bile duct.
3.   Avoid thoracic incisions.
4.   Avoid clamp injury to the renal vessels.
5.   Match the weight of donor and recipient within 20%.
6.   Preserve as much length of the supra- and infrahepatic vena cava, portal vein and hepatic artery as possible.

❍   **What is the most difficult anastomosis to perform in liver transplantation?**

The suprahepatic caval anastomosis.

❍   **What is the best sequence of anastomosis to remove the cold perfusate and prevent systemic hyperthermia and heparinization in liver transplantation?**

The suprahepatic caval, followed by the portal vein, inferior hepatic caval and, finally, the hepatic artery and inferior vena cava.

❍   **What is the next step after vascular anastomosis?**

Biliary drainage; direct bile duct-to-bile duct anastomosis in adults and choledochojejunostomy in children.

❍   **What are the preferred immunosuppressive agents in liver transplant patients if renal function is poor?**

Antilymphoblast serum and AZ (cyclosporin is omitted).

❍   **When is a radionuclide excretory cholangiogram performed after liver transplantation?**

On postoperative day 3 and then at weekly intervals.

❍   **What does a delay in excretion indicate?**

Hepatocellular damage during death of the graft, technical complications, vascular compromise or rejection.

❍   *How is rejection differentiated from ischemia, viral infection and cholangitis?*

Percutaneous liver biopsy.

❍   **What findings suggest cholangitis?**

PMNs within the portal tracts.

❍ **What is the first indication of primary nonfunction of a liver graft?**

Factor V levels fail to return to normal.

❍ **What are the most common causes of encephalopathy following liver transplantation?**

Gastrointestinal bleeding or other protein loads and hepatic coma secondary to cerebral edema and increased intracranial pressure.

❍ **Why is adequate venous access so critical in patients undergoing liver transplantation?**

Because liver transplantation is associated with major volume losses secondary to coagulopathies.

❍ *A 50 year old male, status-post liver transplant, has a rapidly rising serum bilirubin, elevated transaminases, hyperkalemia, hypoglycemia and coagulopathy. What is the most likely diagnosis?*

Thrombotic occlusion of the hepatic artery or portal vein.

❍ **What is the 5-year survival following liver transplantation?**

Greater than 65%.

❍ **What New York Heart Association (NYHA) class indicates need for cardiac transplantation?**

Class III or IV.

❍ **What is the end-stage pathology of cardiomyopathy?**

Dilated cardiac chambers, myocardial degeneration and fibrosis.

❍ **What is the etiology of ischemic cardiomyopathy?**

Viral infection.

❍ **T/F: Patients with idiopathic cardiomyopathy are usually young, otherwise healthy, patients.**

True.

❍ **What are the requirements for designating a patient as Status I by the United Network for Organ Sharing (UNOS)?**

The patient must require intravenous pressors or inotropic agents, an intraaortic balloon pump, respiratory support or a ventricular support device and must require ICU care.

❍ **T/F: All patients requiring a cardiac transplant who are less than 6 months of age are automatically UNOS Status I.**

True.

❍ **Following a median sternotomy, what is the first step in donor cardiectomy?**

Ligation of the SVC and division of the IVC and pulmonary veins.

❍ **What perfusate is used to preserve the donor heart?**

A hyperkalemic cardioplegia solution.

O   **What is the proper order of anastamosis in cardiac transplantation?**

The left atrium, followed by the right atrium, pulmonary arteries and, finally, the aorta.

O   **T/F: The sinus node of the donor heart becomes the dominant pacemaker.**

True.

O   **What is the most common regimen of immunosuppression following cardiac transplantation?**

Triple therapy with oral cyclosporine, AZ and prednisone.

O   **What drugs are used in rescue therapy for cardiac rejection?**

Cytolytic agents (OKT3, ATG and ALG).

O   **What biopsy findings suggest Grade 2 cardiac rejection?**

Focal infiltrates with myocyte necrosis.

O   **What signs and symptoms are associated with cardiac rejection?**

Malaise, fatigue, dyspnea/orthopnea, tachycardia, a ventricular gallop, rales and edema.

O   **What is the treatment of choice for most episodes of cardiac rejection?**

Prednisone.

O   **What is the 5-year survival rate following cardiac transplantation?**

70%.

O   **What is the 30-day mortality rate following cardiac transplantation?**

10%.

O   **What are the most common cardiac causes of early mortality in cardiac transplant patients?**

Poor donor selection, poor donor preservation and prohibitive pulmonary hypertension.

O   **T/F: Graft coronary artery disease (CAD) is often treated with CABG or angioplasty.**

False.

O   **What was the cause of death in most patients receiving lung transplants in the 1960's?**

Dehiscence at the bronchial anastamosis.

O   **What is the most appropriate type of transplant for patients with end-stage Eisenmenger's disease?**

A heart-lung transplant.

O   **What are the indications for double-lung transplantation?**

Cystic fibrosis, bronchiectasis, pulmonary hypertension, correctable congenital defects and emphysema.

O   **Where are the pulmonary veins and pulmonary artery divided in lung transplantation?**

In the hilum.

O   **How is CMV lung disease in a transplanted lung established?**

By finding inclusion bodies in lung tissue obtained by transbronchial biopsy.

O   **What are the key technical factors in heart-lung transplantation?**

Good hemostasis of the middle mediastinum and protection of both phrenic nerves, both vagus nerves and the recurrent nerve.

O   **What is the maintenance immunosuppression following heart-lung transplantation?**

Triple therapy with cyclosporine, AZ and prednisone.

O   **What is the initial treatment for Grade 2 or greater lung rejection?**

An oral or intravenous steroid boost. Refractory rejection is treated with a cytolytic agent.

O   **What is the treatment of choice for patients with severe ventilation/perfusion (V/Q) mismatch following lung transplantation?**

Extracorporeal membrane oxygenation (ECMO).

O   **What biopsy findings are associated with chronic vascular rejection?**

Fibrointimal thickening of the arteries and veins.

O   **What is the 1-year survival rate for heart-lung transplant recipients?**

64%.

O   **What are the most common causes of chronic renal failure?**

Polycystic kidney disease, glomerulonephritis, pyelonephritis and other systemic diseases such as diabetes, systemic lupus erythematosis and Wegner's granulomatosis.

O   **What are the indications for renal dialysis?**

Hyperkalemia, acidosis, fluid overload, symptomatic uremia, drug overdose treatable via dialysis

O   **What are the absolute contraindications to renal transplantation?**

Active infection or malignancy that cannot be brought under control.

O   **What is the success rate for matched renal transplants between siblings?**

95%.

O   **How long can donor kidneys be stored?**

48 to 72 hours.

O   **What is the standard immunosuppressive management following renal transplantation?**

Cyclosporine, AZ and prednisone.

❍   **What is the differential diagnosis for early anuria following renal transplantation?**

Hypovolemia, thrombosis of the renal artery or vein, hyperacute rejection, compression of the kidney or obstruction to urine flow, ATN.

❍   **What is the treatment of choice for urinary extravasation following renal transplantation?**

Re-exploration with reimplantation of the ureter.

AMPUTATION PEARLS

Any fool can cut off a leg - it takes a surgeon to save one.
George C. Ross

○ **What are the vascular indications for amputation?**

Severe arterial insufficiency without bypass target and gangrene.

○ **What is the most common indication for amputation in the United States?**

Peripheral vascular disease (PVD).

○ **T/F: Patients with an above the knee amputation (AKA) expend twice the energy to ambulate as those with a below the knee (BKA) amputation.**

True.

○ **How much of a stump is required for a BKA prosthesis?**

2 inches.

○ **What determines the healing ability of an amputation stump?**

The adequacy of the nutritional blood flow to the skin.

○ **What are the general classes of amputation?**

The standard or conventional amputation, the osteomyoplastic or myodesis amputation and the provisional or open (guillotine) amputation.

○ **What is the operative mortality for amputations performed for trauma, isolated tumor or infection?**

Less than 3%.

○ **What is the most common indication for lower extremity amputation?**

Ischemia.

○ **What type of amputation is associated with the highest healing rates in patients with PVD?**

An AKA.

○ **What is the most common approach for a transmetatarsal amputation?**

A racquet incision.

○ **What is involved in proper postoperative care following amputation?**

Compression dressing followed by elastic dressings to avoid stump edema, splinting of the stump, exercise, proper positioning and early rehabilitation.

❍   **What is the treatment of choice when infection compromises the plantar skin flap of a transmetatarsal amputation?**

A midtarsal amputation.

❍   **What are the major functional advantages of a BKA over an AKA?**

A BKA provides the ability for a more functional prosthesis, easier ambulation, decreased energy expenditure and decreased incidence of phantom pain.

❍   **T/F: The talus is preserved in a Syme amputation.**

False.

❍   **T/F: Ischemic rigor of the calf muscles is a contraindication to BKA.**

True.

❍   **What are the disadvantages of knee disarticulation?**

The end of the stump is bulky and has bony prominences that make prosthesis fitting more difficult.

❍   **What are the indications for a hip disarticulation?**

Bone tumors, soft tissue tumors, chronic decubitus ulcers unresponsive to reconstructive procedures and extensive traumatic injury.

❍   **What are the advantages of wrist disarticulation over more proximal amputations?**

It preserves length and provides better control of prosthesis.

❍   **T/F: A very short below-elbow amputation is preferable to an above-elbow amputation.**

True.

❍   **What is the survival rate following traumatic hemipelvectomy?**

Less than 50%.

❍   **What are the requirements for a lower extremity prosthesis?**

A socket to interface with the residual limb (stump) and a suspension device.

❍   **What is the most critical aspect of a lower extremity prosthesis?**

A properly fitting and comfortable socket across which residual limb forces are transmitted.

❍   **What is the most common type of prosthetic socket used for an AK amputee?**

The quadrilateral total-contact socket.

❍   **What is the most common indication for an upper extremity amputation?**

Trauma.

○   **T/F: In digital phalanx amputations, the volar flap should be longer than the dorsal flap.**

True.

○   **T/F: A patient with an AKA is more likely to develop a postoperative complication than a patient with a BKA.**

False.

Suggested Text Readings for General Surgeons

ACS Surgery, Principles and Practice. Souba, et. al., WebMD Professional Publishing, 2004.

Advancements in the diagnosis of acute appendicitis in children and adolescents. Blab E, Kohlhuber U, Tillawi S, Schweitzer M, Stangl G, Ogris E, Rokitansky A. Eur J Pediatr Surg. 2004 Dec;14(6):404-9.

Advanced Trauma Life Support. Educational course and text provided by American College of Surgeons. Visit www.facs.org for course details and sign up information.

Chemoradiotherapy for head and neck cancer: current status and perspectives. Kawashima M. Int J Clin Oncol. 2004 Dec;9(6):421-34.

Current Surgical Therapy, 8th Edition. Cameron. C.V. Mosby, 2004.

Essentials of General Surgery. 3rd Edition. Lawrence. Lippincott Williams & Wilkens, 2000.

Principles of Surgery, 8th Edition., Schwartz, et. al., McGraw Hill Publishing, 2004.

Surgery : Scientific Principles and Practice, 3rd Edition. Greenfield, et. al., Lippincott, Williams, and Wilkins, 2001.

Surgical Critical Care. O'Donnell, et. al., Kluwer Academic Publishers, 2001.

Thoracic Surgery, 2nd Edition. Pearson, et. al., Churchill Livingstone, 2002.

Vascular Surgery, 5th Edition. Rutherford. Saunders, 2000.